Living Your Best

WITH

Early-Stage

Alzheimer's

alzheimer's association

Desert Southwest Chapter
Northern Arizona Region
3111 Clearwater Drive, Suite A
Prescott AZ 86305

Lisa Snyder, MSW, LCSW

University of California-San Diego
Shiley-Marcos Alzheimer's Disease Research Center

Foreword by Douglas Galasko, MD
Director, Shiley-Marcos Alzheimer's Disease Research Center

SUNRISE
River Press

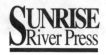

Sunrise River Press
39966 Grand Avenue
North Branch, MN 55056
Phone: 651-277-1400 or 800-895-4585
Fax: 651-277-1203
www.sunriseriverpress.com

Edit by Karin Craig
Layout by Monica Seiberlich

ISBN 978-1-934716-03-8
Item No. SRP603

Library of Congress Cataloging-in-Publication Data

Snyder, Lisa.
  Living your best with early-stage Alzheimer's : an essential guide / by Lisa Snyder.
    p. cm.
  Includes bibliographical references and index.
  ISBN 978-1-934716-03-8
  1. Alzheimer's disease--Popular works. I. Title.
  RC523.2.S6449 2010
  616.8'31--dc22
                            2009047788

Printed in USA
10 9 8 7 6 5 4 3 2

Contents

Foreword....................5
Acknowledgments....................9
Introduction....................10

Part 1: An Overview of Alzheimer's

CHAPTER 1: What Is Alzheimer's Disease?....................13
CHAPTER 2: Understanding Your Reactions to the Diagnosis....................23
CHAPTER 3: Symptoms You Could Experience....................30

Part 2: Your Family and Friends

CHAPTER 4: Talking with Others about Alzheimer's....................41
CHAPTER 5: Taking Care of Family Relationships....................48
CHAPTER 6: The Unique Concerns of Young-Onset Alzheimer's Families..56
CHAPTER 7: Maintaining Friendships and Creating New Ones....................66
CHAPTER 8: Strategies for Effective Communication with Friends and Family....................72

Part 3: Daily Living

CHAPTER 9: Helpful Tips for Managing Memory Loss....................80
CHAPTER 10: Dealing Effectively with Other Symptoms....................90
CHAPTER 11: Improving the Safety of Your Home Environment....................97
CHAPTER 12: Making Decisions about Driving....................104
CHAPTER 13: If You Live Alone....................112

Part 4: Coping With Alzheimer's

CHAPTER 14: Understanding and Managing Your Feelings....................121
CHAPTER 15: The Benefits of Support Groups for You and Your Family...133
CHAPTER 16: Learning to Accept Help When You Need It....................142
CHAPTER 17: Finding Meaningful Activities....................150
CHAPTER 18: Speaking Your Mind Through Advocacy....................163

Part 5: Maintaining Your Emotional and Physical Health

CHAPTER 19: Boosting Your Physical and Mental Health
Through Exercise 171

CHAPTER 20: The Benefits of Mental Stimulation.................................178

CHAPTER 21: Food for Thought: The Value of Good Nutrition.............185

CHAPTER 22: Maintaining Hope and a Sense of Humor.......................192

CHAPTER 23: Taking Care of Your Care Partner 200

Part 6: Plans to Make Now and For the Future

CHAPTER 24: Finding and Using Available Community Resources 209

CHAPTER 25: Creating and Communicating with Your
Healthcare Team 215

CHAPTER 26: Helpful Legal, Financial and Long-Term Planning.............223

CHAPTER 27: Maintaining an Ongoing Quality of Life.........................232

Part 7: Hopeful Possibilities in Treatment and Research

CHAPTER 28: Progress and Trends in Treatment and Care 239

CHAPTER 29: Complementary and Alternative Therapies.......................247

CHAPTER 30: Research Brings Hope for the Future...............................256

Helpful Resources 265

References..268

Index 276

Foreword

Lifespan has increased dramatically in the United States and Westernized countries in the past 100 years, and more people are able to lead active lives into their eighties and beyond. However, the downside of this success is that diseases associated with aging are also increasing. One of the most important of these is Alzheimer's disease, which together with other dementias affects over 5 million people in the United States at present, a number which is projected to rise. These estimates are largely based on studies of people aged 65 or older, and we have a less clear idea of how many people may be affected with dementia at a younger age. The costs associated with Alzheimer's disease are enormous, and they provide an indirect index of how the progressive cognitive changes make people increasingly dependent on others.

On a personal level, Alzheimer's disease attacks what are our most precious resources: our memories. During the course of the disease, people progress from initially requiring reminders or supervision to carry out complex activities, to needing greater degrees of help, eventually becoming dependent for basic daily activities and functions. The impact of Alzheimer's disease extends to family members and friends, who need to acquire a complex set of skills to function effectively as caregivers and supporters. Although Alzheimer's disease challenges key aspects of our personal abilities, the responses of making the most of preserved cognitive functions, establishing a comprehensive care plan and maintaining a supportive and nurturing social and physical environment once someone has this diagnosis can help greatly to mitigate the effects of dementia.

A burgeoning amount of information about brain function in aging and dementia is now available through books, Web sites, and community organizations. Even within this accessible pool of expert advice, there are gaps and less well-surveyed areas. This book covers one of them: the questions associated with early-stage Alzheimer's disease. The increase in awareness about memory changes and Alzheimer's disease has led to many people undergoing evaluation and receiving a diagnosis at an early stage, when symptoms are relatively mild. This presents opportunities, because the person who has received the diagnosis is better able to participate in planning and decision-making, and to understand the choices more clearly. Among the most frequently voiced concerns are how (and where) to obtain an accurate diagnosis, how to deal with social and financial questions—for example, what to do regarding work and driving, and where to identify the most appropriate social resources, such as community or support groups that tailor to the needs of people who have a degree of forgetfulness but may be largely independent.

Lisa Snyder has written this timely book as a guide to empower patients, and to help them to work with family, friends, community organizations, and healthcare providers to navigate through these questions and many others. There is a wealth of information on measures to maintain resilience, preserve general and physical health, and to seek enjoyment and identify appropriate and meaningful activities. Interactions with friends and family often change once someone is diagnosed as having Alzheimer's disease, and there are chapters that suggest ways to improve communication and preserve relationships and social networks.

The original patient described by Alois Alzheimer was a woman whose symptoms began in her fifties. For many years, researchers divided Alzheimer's disease into 'presenile' and 'senile' types, based solely on age at onset. This concept did not hold up upon further study: it turned out that, regardless of age at onset, the same types of plaques and tangles that Alzheimer originally identified were always present in the brain. Although Alzheimer's disease is now thought of as a continuum, there are notable differences, problems and challenges when it manifests in someone younger than 65. Again, the material in this book contains a summary of the special issues and concerns that may relate to people with younger onset of Alzheimer's disease, and a helpful list of resources is provided.

I have had the pleasure of interacting with Lisa Snyder for over 20 years, in her capacity as a Social Worker at the University of California, San Diego's Alzheimer's Disease Research Center. Lisa's reassurance, compassion and skilled guidance have helped many families at our Center negotiate the rugged terrain of coping with dementia. Her enthusiasm for ensuring that patients and families receive the best advice available and are knowledgeable about Alzheimer's and the specific resources they should be able to find in the community has led her to establish or improve on many of those resources. In particular, Lisa has developed support groups and activity programs for patients in the early stages of Alzheimer's disease, and for early-onset dementia. Several of Lisa's innovative programs aimed at increasing social stimulation for patients with Alzheimer's disease have proven to be extremely popular and successful, and she has collaborated in establishing similar programs throughout San Diego County and elsewhere. Through books, newsletters and talks, Lisa has spread the word about providing a high standard of care and enriching the lives of people with Alzheimer's.

A particular cause of Lisa's is that patients should not be forgotten or ignored: although they may have cognitive difficulties, they still have voices. People who interact with someone with Alzheimer's disease need to acknowledge this and make the most of them as people, and Lisa is a persuasive advocate for having the patient continue to live as fully as possible during the course of the disease. Lisa has developed a special facility for communicating with patients and their families. This has infused the style of this book, as it is directed to the patient with Alzheimer's disease, and is written in a highly accessible manner. Someone with memory or cognitive problems should be able to understand the clear exposition that this book provides, and will benefit from reviewing the questions at the end of each chapter. The material is comprehensive and current enough that caregivers or family members of any patient with dementia can benefit.

Our main hope for the future is research. This book provides a succinct coverage of standard medical treatment, and advice on the important—and often confusing—topics of exercise, cognitive stimulation and nutritional supplements. Current research efforts regarding new methods to diagnose Alzheimer's disease and new forms of treatment are outlined. Critical information to guide people in their decisions to participate in research studies, including the important topic of clinical trials of new medications. This book will be valuable beyond its intent as a resource for patients with the earliest stages of Alzheimer's disease; it is readily accessible for caregivers, families, and care providers to improve the roles they play in forming a collaborative caring team.

Douglas Galasko, MD
Director, Shiley-Marcos Alzheimer's Disease Research Center
University of California, San Diego

Acknowledgments

I am indebted to many dearly valued friends, colleagues, and family members who gave generously of their time, expertise, and insight to review sections of this book. My sincere gratitude to Dr. Paul Aisen, Dr. Jody Corey-Bloom, Judy Filippoff, Dr. Douglas Galasko, Patricia Hunter, Dr. Cecily Jenkins, Kathy McClelland, Paulette Michaud, Darby Morhardt, Dr. Mike Raffi, Dr. David Salmon, Jennifer Snyder, Mike Splaine, Becky Wong, and Robyn Yale. My husband, Jeff Irwin, steadfastly sustained me throughout this project with his astute feedback and enduring encouragement.

Since 1992, I have had the privilege of co-facilitating support groups for people with early-stage Alzheimer's and their care partners where a great deal of wisdom has been shared over the years. I do not have permission to name each of you individually, but please know that I am humbled by the insights, ingenuity, and humanity exchanged in these meetings, and sincerely grateful to those support group participants who gave invaluable feedback as this manuscript took shape.

Many thanks to Dan Kuhn for recommending me to Sunrise River Press during their search for an author to write this book. Karin Craig, my editor, was exceptionally gracious, patient, and thoughtful throughout the conceptualization and fine-tuning of the manuscript. Barbara Harold and Josh Brown attended to additional editing and Connie Nordrum and Monica Seiberlich to design and layout.

Several individuals with Alzheimer's are quoted throughout this text. I am deeply appreciative of the wisdom that they contribute to this book and to my life. Over the years, so many people with Alzheimer's have inspired me to try to live my best and embrace each day that I am given. I hope that this book can provide some encouragement and guidance in return.

❀ Introduction

The aim of this book is to provide an encouraging and informative guide for people living with early-stage Alzheimer's or a related disorder. Although there are numerous books written to address the needs and concerns of families or care partners, there is little written directly for the benefit of those who are living day to day with the experience of memory loss and other challenging changes. As a result, persons with Alzheimer's can feel left out of the opportunity to gain valuable information, coping skills, and methods for living effectively with symptoms. Although there are a growing number of pamphlets, booklets, and personal narratives, written for or by people with Alzheimer's on a variety of relevant issues, this book organizes much useful information and advice into one comprehensive guide.

It is vital to know that there are creative and constructive ways to manage early-stage Alzheimer's. Through respectful communication with others, as well as strategic and resourceful coping, you can maximize your abilities and move forward with your life. This book also serves as a guide for family members, friends, or professionals who want to learn how to be of help to you, and partner with you so that you can better meet any challenges together.

How to Use This Book

Living Your Best With Early-Stage Alzheimer's is organized into 30 short chapters, each addressing a specific issue. This format is based on feedback from people with Alzheimer's, who say that they often prefer to read brief chunks of information so they can more effectively remember or process the content. The multiple chapters also allow you to choose pages to read as needed, based on a current need or concern. Thus, it is not necessary to read the book from cover to cover. Rather, each chapter stands on its own and can be read in whatever order is desired, or as often as needed for a refresher. The chapters are clustered in seven parts that are organized according to themes common to the early stages of Alzheimer's.

Each chapter ends with discussion questions that are included to build dialogue between people with Alzheimer's and their loved ones. Frequently, individuals and families do not feel comfortable discussing these sensitive topics or do not know where to begin. Discussion questions can also be posed to yourself as a means of thinking through the chapter material or used in support group or education meetings to prompt group conversations and learning.

Suggestions relevant to each chapter topic follow the discussion questions and offer constructive advice or practical steps to take. Not all suggestions will be meaningful to you or workable for everyone, but they are offered for consideration so that you can take action when you choose to or when needed.

The Value of Learning from People with Alzheimer's

For more than two decades, I have had the privilege of assisting thousands of individuals and families in navigating the often confusing terrain of early-stage Alzheimer's through facilitating weekly early-stage support groups, providing individual and family counseling, editing an international early-stage newsletter, and engaging in daily phone and email conversations with people with Alzheimer's from all around the country and occasionally, the world. I have listened to the needs, feelings, and concerns of these individuals and families, and I have learned almost everything in this book by creating trusting spaces where their insights and wisdom could be revealed and shared with others. As such, this book is infused with direct quotes from people with Alzheimer's who helped guide the content and reinforce the importance of hearing their voices and listening to their messages.

When quotes in this book have been published elsewhere, they are cited using the same name that was attributed to the speaker or writer of the published quote. If the quote is from my personal conversation with the speaker or from a support group meeting session, I have used the authentic first name only or the complete name based on the speaker's permission. In those instances when I have a quote documented from personal conversation or published literature where there is no name attached to the quote or I do not have permission to use a name, I have used the phrase "one woman" or "one man" to identify the speaker rather than use a fictitious name.

A primary objective of this book is to help ease the fear and isolation that can accompany an Alzheimer's diagnosis by providing open discussion and problem solving about sensitive yet common concerns. Whether you are a person with Alzheimer's, a loved one, or a professional in the field, I hope this book will help you to develop tools to shape your own experience and inspire you to share your perspectives with others. There are many paths to living your best with Alzheimer's, and we are all made better by our collective efforts to help one another along the way.

Chapter One

What is Alzheimer's Disease?

Many people have heard the word Alzheimer's on television or the radio, or have seen it in newspapers and magazines. If you are reading this book, the word has more personal significance for you now. Although each person can be affected differently, a basic understanding of Alzheimer's is the first step in learning how to live with its symptoms effectively.

Alzheimer's disease is a brain disorder that begins gradually and progresses over time. The course of Alzheimer's can span 2 to 20 years, with great variability in symptoms and rate of change. The main symptom is a decline in memory and thinking that results in difficulty performing routine activities, such as keeping

> *An early diagnosis can help you develop effective strategies for managing symptoms and moving forward with life.*

appointments, managing a checkbook, or fulfilling work obligations. Although these changes can be mild in the early stages of Alzheimer's, they become more significant over time and result in greater challenges with your thinking processes, daily activities, and ability to take care of yourself.

Changes in memory and other areas of thinking are due to the death of nerve cells in the brain (neurons) and the breakdown of the connections between them (synapses) that enable the brain to function. Doctors now have greater ability to recognize the earliest signs of Alzheimer's and can often make a diagnosis when symptoms are still in the beginning stages. While it may be hard to believe that you have Alzheimer's, an early diagnosis can be key to helping you and your loved ones develop effective strategies for managing symptoms and moving forward with life.

Why Did You Get Alzheimer's?

For most people, there is no clear reason why they develop Alzheimer's, but scientists have identified a number of risk factors. Advanced age, family history, specific genes, female gender, significant head injury, and certain other medical conditions are the greatest risk factors. Alzheimer's is a worldwide condition, sparing no country or group of people.

The risk of developing Alzheimer's grows dramatically with age, doubling every 5 years beyond age 65. Research indicates that while one in ten people over the age of 65 have Alzheimer's, up to half of those over age 85 are affected. While some scientists theorize that anyone who lives long enough will eventually develop Alzheimer's, most agree that Alzheimer's disease is distinct from normal aging, and methods should be found to prevent or treat its destructive impact on the brain.

A family history with one or more parents or siblings with Alzheimer's also increases your risk of developing the disease. Scientists have discovered gene mutations on chromosomes 1, 14, and 21 that can cause Alzheimer's in people diagnosed at a particularly young age (generally under age 60), but these genetic mutations account for fewer than 5 percent of all Alzheimer's cases. Many people who develop Alzheimer's earlier in life do not have these mutations.

Other genes have been linked to an increased risk of developing Alzheimer's later in life, but they may not be wholly responsible for causing onset. For example, apolipoprotein E (APOE) is a protein that helps to carry cholesterol and fat in the blood. One form, or allele, of this protein, APOE4, is present in up to half of those who develop Alzheimer's after age 60. This allele, also influential in heart disease, may be inherited from one or both parents. Although one can have the APOE4 allele and not develop Alzheimer's, its presence increases the risk. Doctors do not usually recommend being tested for the APOE4 gene because it does not determine for certain if a person will ultimately develop Alzheimer's.

The National Institutes of Health and research institutes around the world are conducting numerous genome-wide association studies (GWAS) to map a wide array of genes specifically associated with Alzheimer's and related disorders. Many new genes have already been discovered and are leading to hopeful avenues for detection, treatments, and prevention of these conditions. At present, researchers do not recommend that individuals seek testing for these risk factor genes because their role in the development of Alzheimer's is still unclear.

Women are at increased risk for developing Alzheimer's largely due to their longer life span. Some scientists argue that diminished estrogen levels after menopause may play a role in making the brain more susceptible to Alzheimer changes. Estrogen therapy, however, is currently not recommended for Alzheimer's prevention.

Medical conditions that increase risk for Alzheimer's include diabetes, Down syndrome, heart disease, hypertension (high blood pressure) vascular disease (strokes), as well as a history of head injury, including loss of consciousness or multiple blows to the head. Some evidence suggests that chronic untreated depression may make the brain more vulnerable to Alzheimer's, as can a low level of education.

People with one or more risk factors may be more likely to develop Alzheimer's, but many never do. Likewise, many people who do develop Alzheimer's do not have any known risk factors and question how this could happen. While it is common to ask, "Why me?" in response to a diagnosis, it is important to know that you have not been singled out and are not to blame. More than 5 million people in the United States and an estimated 35 million people worldwide have Alzheimer's disease. You are not alone.

Why You Have Memory Loss

The brain is a complex organ, and scientists have long attempted to understand its workings. In the early 1900s, the German physician Alois Alzheimer was curious about the cause of significant and progressive memory loss and personality changes in one of his patients. When this patient died, Dr. Alzheimer performed an autopsy of her brain. He discovered a dramatic loss of her nerve cells due to large numbers of what came to be known as *neurofibrillary tangles* and *neuritic plaques*. These destructive microscopic plaques and tangles are composed of abnormal protein deposits in the brain and are the hallmark of Alzheimer's disease. Tangles are made up of *tau* protein and get lodged inside the nerve cell. Plaques form outside the nerve cell and are made up of *amyloid* protein. Although scientists continue to debate the effects of plaques and tangles on the brain, many think these protein deposits are at the root of Alzheimer's-related brain changes.

The brain is made up of numerous regions, each responsible for various functions of thinking, feeling, and movement. Alzheimer's disease usually starts in the hippocampus, a region of the brain that is primarily responsible for receiving new information and temporarily storing it, and then facilitating its move into other areas of the brain for long-term storage. As plaques and tangles begin to form in the hippocampus, the brain's ability to store new information is disrupted. However, old information that was stored throughout the brain prior to the onset of Alzheimer's may be unaffected for quite some time. That is why it may be difficult for you to remember new information, but you can vividly remember something that happened in your childhood.

How Your Doctor Diagnoses Alzheimer's

Alzheimer's is a form of dementia. Dimentia is a general category of conditions that result in a decline in thinking abilities. There are more than 70 different causes of dementia, but Alzheimer's disease is the most common type. Your physician must rule out any other kind of dementia or cause for your memory loss before making a diagnosis of Alzheimer's. During your evaluation, it is common for a doctor to talk with your spouse or a close family member or friend who can give a detailed description of the onset of your memory or functional problems. This is because memory loss can affect your own ability to accurately recall details about your symptoms. This discussion is usually followed by a physical and neurological exam.

During this exam, your physician conducts a "mental status test" to help evaluate your overall thinking abilities. Just as a thermometer reading can alert a physician to fever in the body, the mental status exam is a tool that can alert a physician to potential difficulty in brain function. In these tests, you are asked to complete a set of mental and physical tasks associated with various brain functions such as language, memory, problem solving, and spatial abilities (the ability to judge distance and perspective). A diagnosis of Alzheimer's requires that you have abnormal changes in memory and in at least one or more of these other areas of thinking. These changes must interfere with your ability to carry out routine tasks or daily activities.

A brain scan is often recommended in order to rule out strokes, tumors, or brain changes attributable to other conditions and to look for patterns consistent with Alzheimer's. Blood work helps to rule out kidney, liver, or thyroid problems, nutritional deficiencies, or other metabolic imbalances. You may also be asked about your mood, because depression can cause changes in thinking and memory. Some physicians order a lumbar puncture to rule out certain brain infections or to look for elevated levels of a specific protein associated with Alzheimer's. There is currently no specific test that can diagnosis Alzheimer's disease with absolute certainty other than a brain biopsy that reveals the hallmark plaques and tangles. Physicians can, however, achieve at least 90 percent accuracy in diagnosing Alzheimer's by performing a thorough evaluation that does not include this invasive brain surgery procedure.

When the Diagnosis is Not Alzheimer's

You may hear or read about Alzheimer's *and related disorders*. Related disorders refers to other conditions that result in memory loss or changes in your thinking and behavior. The most common related disorders are Mild Cognitive Impairment (considered a likely precursor to Alzheimer's); Vascular Dementia (a result of one or more strokes); Frontotemporal Dementia (often involves significant changes in personality or behavior); or Lewy Body Dementia (usually includes physical symptoms of Parkinson's disease).

If you have been diagnosed with one of these related disorders, you may not identify with all of the symptoms associated with Alzheimer's, or you may have some other symptoms unique to your own condition. All of these related disorders have many issues in common, though, and regardless of your specific diagnosis, this book aims to address these shared issues and concerns.

Principles for a Dignified Diagnosis

The evaluation and diagnosis of Alzheimer's or a related disorder can be a stressful process. People with Alzheimer's report varied experiences with their doctors and how the diagnosis was or was not given. Some feel the diagnosis was presented clearly or compassionately while others have less favorable experiences. Some may learn about their presumed diagnosis in unexpected ways. Harold Seiden writes about his experience being prescribed Aricept (a treatment for Alzheimer's) without any awareness of his diagnosis:

> "In retrospect, I experienced a common problem that occurs with dementia and Alzheimer's patients and their doctors when first diagnosed with the condition. Should the doctor give the diagnosis to the patient and his family or not? Should the condition be given a name to the patient? Being an early-stage dementia patient, I was surprised to see a New York Times ad for Aricept, stating it's a treatment for Alzheimer's. This is not the way I should have gotten the news of my condition."[1]

Through a series of nationwide town hall meetings with families facing early-stage Alzheimer's, the Alzheimer's Association learned that many individuals experienced challenges getting a thorough evaluation and diagnosis and had dissatisfying interactions with the medical community. As a result, the Association worked with an advisory group of people with Alzheimer's to create the *Principles for a Dignified Diagnosis*.[2] The following principles were written by persons with Alzheimer's on how to improve the experience.

Talk to me directly, the person with dementia.

I am the person with the disease, and though my loved ones will also be affected, I am the person who needs to know first.

Tell the truth.

Even if you don't have all the answers, be honest about what you do know and why you believe it to be so.

Test early.

Helping me get an accurate diagnosis as soon as possible gives me more time to cope and live to my fullest potential and to get information about appropriate clinical trials.

Take my concerns seriously, regardless of my age.

Age may be the biggest risk factor for Alzheimer's, but Alzheimer's is not a normal part of aging. Don't discount my concerns because I am old. At the same time, don't forget that Alzheimer's can also affect people in their 40s, 50s, and 60s.

Deliver the news in plain but sensitive language.

This may be one of the most important things I ever hear. Please use language that I can understand and is sensitive to how this may make me feel.

Coordinate with other care providers.

I may be seeing more than one specialist. It is important that you talk to my other providers to ensure you all have the information so that changes can be identified early on and I don't have to repeat any tests unnecessarily.

Explain the purpose of different tests and what you hope to learn.

Testing can be very physically and emotionally challenging. It would help me to know what the purpose of the test is, how long it will take, and what you expect to learn from the process. I would also appreciate the option of breaks during longer tests and an opportunity to ask questions.

Give me tools for living with this disease.

Please don't give me my diagnosis and then leave me alone to confront it. I need to know what will happen to me, and I need to know not only about medical treatment options but also what support is available through the Alzheimer's Association and other resources in my community.

Work with me on a plan for healthy living.

Medication may help modify some of my neurological symptoms, but I am also interested in other recommendations for keeping myself as healthy as possible through diet, exercise, and social engagement.

Recognize that I am an individual and the way I experience this disease is unique.

This disease affects each person in different ways and at a different pace. Please be sure to couch your explanation of how this disease may change my life with this in mind.

Alzheimer's is a journey, not a destination.

Treatment doesn't end with the writing of a prescription. Please continue to be an advocate—not just for my medical care, but for my quality of life as I continue to live with Alzheimer's.

Principles for a Dignified Diagnosis is available to view and print at www.alz.org and also by request through the Alzheimer's Association.

Learning More About Alzheimer's

Upon hearing the diagnosis "Alzheimer's," many people seek more information and services, hoping to gain knowledge so they can be proactive or cope more effectively. Some people benefit from knowledge and feel empowered by it. Others, however, are overwhelmed or discouraged by too much information about possibilities that may or may not lie ahead.

Pick and choose the information you read carefully based on your own coping style. You may want to select resources that are written specifically for people with Alzheimer's or that are applicable to more early-stage issues. Recognize that your loved ones may have their own interest in seeking educational materials, and be respectful of each other's needs. It is not necessary to try to learn everything there is to know about Alzheimer's immediately. Pace yourself, be selective, and know that more information is always available to you when you need it.

Questions for Discussion

- Did your doctor do a comprehensive workup before diagnosing Alzheimer's?
- Has the doctor talked with you clearly about your diagnosis? How well did he or she follow the *Principles for a Dignified Diagnosis*?
- Do you have any risk factors for Alzheimer's? Are you concerned that something caused it?
- Do you feel you have enough information about Alzheimer's? If not, what information do you need?

Suggestions for Learning More About Alzheimer's

- If you have questions about your diagnosis, ask your doctor to write down the tests that were done during your evaluation and their results. If you do not think you received a thorough evaluation, seek a second opinion. Obtain a copy of *Principles for a Dignified Diagnosis* to share with your doctor at your next appointment.
- Realize that Alzheimer's is found worldwide and there is no clear reason why most people develop the disease. If you are worried about

what might have caused your Alzheimer's, discuss any concerns with your doctor.

- For more information about Alzheimer's, investigate the following national organizations for online and written materials:
  – Alzheimer's Association at 800-272-3900 or www.alz.org
  – Alzheimer's Disease Education and Referral (ADEAR) at 800-438-4380 or www.nia.nih.gov/Alzheimers
  – Alzheimer's Foundation of America (AFA) at 866-232-8484 or www.alzfdn.org
- Consider signing up for these free informative resources:
  – *Perspectives: A Newsletter for Individuals with Alzheimer's or a Related Disorder*, published quarterly by the University of California San Diego Shiley-Marcos Alzheimer's Disease Research Center. Sign up by emailing Lisa Snyder at lsnyder@ucsd.edu.
  – Ageless Designs Alzheimer's News Service—One daily email provides you with informative international news headlines pertaining to Alzheimer's and related disorders and is an excellent way to stay updated about relevant news. Sign up at www.agelessdesign.com.
- Look for classes or support groups specific to early-stage Alzheimer's. The organizations above may be able to refer you to early-stage programs in your community.

Chapter Two

Understanding Your Reactions to the Diagnosis

People with Alzheimer's report a variety of responses to receiving the diagnosis. Some have little memory of the experience. Others may be confused or uncertain about the information because a physician did not discuss the diagnosis with them directly. Some have feelings of disbelief or shock, while others are relieved because they finally have an explanation for their confusing and frightening symptoms. Frequently, however, a diagnosis is met with a mixture of feelings, and it can take time for the news to sink in.

> *"My counselor said, 'It's a bend in the road, not the end of the road' and I think that's right."*

It is Common to Have Some Denial About the Diagnosis

When a person cannot accept the reality of a distressing situation or piece of news, it is often said that he or she is "in denial." Denial may be temporary, or it can continue indefinitely. When diagnosed with Alzheimer's, some people deny that they have a problem because they are not ready or able to accept this information. Denial can give a person some needed time to adjust to the news. In an essay for an Alzheimer's Association newsletter, James Anthony describes a benefit of denial: "A degree of denial is essential. Like somebody drinking hot coffee, we sip the truth of our condition carefully and gently."[1] During a support group meeting, a man who was diagnosed with Alzheimer's in his early 50s says, "I'm interested in this idea of denial. I think denial is helpful sometimes. You don't want to be carrying this all of the time."[2] Others may minimize problems due to fear of distressing their loved ones or concerns about becoming a burden.

Some people deny they have Alzheimer's because of the images they associate with the disease. The media more often portrays people with advanced Alzheimer's and gives less attention to those who are only mildly affected and functioning well. If your thoughts or images of Alzheimer's are of people with advanced symptoms, you may feel frightened and think, "That can't be me!" Others may support your denial by saying that you "seem just fine" and that "everyone forgets." Gerrit says, "Some of my friends still don't believe me because I don't fit into their idea of what Alzheimer's looks like. They don't think there's anything wrong with me."[3] Because doctors are more skilled now at making a diagnosis when symptoms are mild, you may hear the term "early-stage" Alzheimer's as a way of describing your condition. Sometimes doctors are reluctant to be direct about the diagnosis for fear of upsetting the patient, and this can contribute to a person's denial, as well.

Some people may deny they have Alzheimer's because they fear a loss of independence or control. In his book, *My Journey Into Alzheimer's*, Robert Davis writes:

> "Certainly one of the very real fears felt by anyone with early Alzheimer's disease is the fear of failure. I live with the imminent dread that one mistake in my daily life will mean another freedom will be taken from me."[4]

You may be concerned that if others know you have Alzheimer's, they will begin to be overprotective or make too many decisions for you. However, persistent denial of Alzheimer's may actually make others more concerned about you. If you are able to acknowledge that you have memory loss or other symptoms, others will feel they can discuss matters more openly with you and involve you in discussions and decision making.

You May Forget That You Forget

Denial is not always within your control. Since memory loss is the primary symptom of Alzheimer's, you may forget that you are forgetful. Alzheimer's-related changes in your thinking can limit your awareness of your symptoms. Dick Tilleli writes:

> "At first, I couldn't fathom the changes in my memory. I didn't know what was happening. And I didn't know why it was happening. I felt that although I wasn't ill, there was something wrong with my brain…I guess I should have felt it coming on, but I don't know that anyone could feel it coming on. It was a slow thing…Sometimes I feel as if I don't have Alzheimer's. In a way I suppose it's good that I don't remember because I'd be angry with myself if I remembered everything that was going on. I think that although I know I have Alzheimer's, I don't know that it's doing me any harm."[5]

James Anthony recalls that he was not aware of his memory loss until others pointed it out to him. He writes, "It is very difficult for a person with Alzheimer's to experience his disease. You cannot experience what you have forgotten."[6] Another man who agreed to participate in an Alzheimer's research program stated matter-of-factly, "My wife says there's a problem, but I'm not aware of it."

While some people with Alzheimer's trust that their doctor or family members are accurate in their observations, others can become defensive at any mention of their memory loss or other symptoms. If you are not aware of a problem or frequently forget that you have one, you must place your trust in those who have observed unusual changes in your thinking or behavior. It is unlikely that your loved ones are making this up, and doctors do not make a diagnosis of Alzheimer's without significant evidence of a problem.

You Could Be Angry at Others

Some people with mild symptoms feel as if others are making a whole lot of fuss about nothing and can become angry during the process of evaluation and diagnosis. In the Canadian video *I Have Alzheimer Disease*, produced by the Alzheimer Society of Belleville, Ron says to his wife:

> "I think I could say that I was mad at you in the beginning because you were the one who took me to the doctor and I had all those tests and then I'm having my brain examined… I kept thinking, 'Why did she do this?' It would be better if I didn't know. That would be foolishness, but that's how things went through my head."[7]

It is normal to feel angry that this is happening to you or to those you love. It is important that you try to direct any angry feelings to Alzheimer's itself, and not to yourself or your loved ones. Many people find that their anger subsides as they make necessary adjustments and learn more effective coping strategies for managing symptoms.

Concerns About Stigma Surrounding the Diagnosis

Some people with Alzheimer's are concerned about the stigma associated with their diagnosis and fear that others could view them with less regard. These concerns can contribute to feelings of shame about your symptoms or attempts to keep the information private. Betty says:

"In the past, people never uttered the word Alzheimer's for fear that they would catch it...It used to be that way around cancer. But now Alzheimer's disease has gotten a lot of media attention, and the symptoms that are described scare people—that we'll walk blindly into a car because we're lost and wandering. It isn't necessarily true but people get an idea. When it comes to Alzheimer's, you're not sure how people will respond to you."[8]

Changes in functional or thinking abilities can lead some to feel left out of mainstream life. When diagnosed with Alzheimer's, Les Dennis described this experience as "marginalization," a feeling of being on the margins of life. He writes:

"I began to understand the concept of marginalization and its relationship to Alzheimer's. Simply put, get up and do what you can or you will fade, fairly quickly. As I tried this out with myself, then my children, it seemed to work. You remain someone."[9]

Although he may find it more challenging to be the person he has always been, Les has made an important decision to not give in to stigma or feelings of diminishment and is determined to stay engaged in life.

As public awareness about Alzheimer's grows, there is greater understanding about this disability. Education greatly reduces stigma, and more people with Alzheimer's are taking part in these efforts to increase awareness and reduce marginalization (see Chapter 18).

The Diagnosis May Be Frightening or Shocking

Many people have frightening associations with the word Alzheimer's and can't imagine how they will learn to live with the condition. Bernie Shapiro recalls the moment he was diagnosed. He writes in an Alzheimer's Association newsletter:

"I was devastated, in shock, speechless. I could not believe that I could have Alzheimer's. I am in excellent health, and truly believed that I would have a long and healthy life. I was angry, depressed, felt suicidal, and hated the world. After experiencing this myriad of emotions, I calmed down and realized that there is still a world out there for me to participate in."[10]

It is common to experience a range of feelings when you receive difficult news. Some people recall feeling that their life was suddenly over when they heard the diagnosis, or they may have difficult memories of a parent of grandparent who had Alzheimer's. If you have a family history of Alzheimer's, it is important to understand that each person's experience with Alzheimer's is different. Ongoing advances in treatment and services could afford you access to types of care that were not available to your parent or grandparent.

Sometimes the Diagnosis is a Relief

Many people with Alzheimer's and their loved ones experience increased stress and tension in their relationships prior to the diagnosis. Memory loss and other symptoms can affect your mood, abilities, and routines, and there may be a phase when everyone is puzzled and aggravated by these unusual changes. A diagnosis can actually be a relief because it provides an explanation for the changes and a medical reason for the symptoms you are experiencing. A diagnosis can bring more clarity to confusing circumstances, and everyone can begin to learn more effective ways of dealing with problems. One man says:

"I didn't know why I was acting these ways I didn't understand. I just couldn't seem to get a handle on things. The diagnosis gave me just about as good a reason as you can get for my confusion. It's not such a mystery now and we're really managing better... My counselor said, 'It's a bend in the road, not the end of the road,' and I think that's right."

Reactions to the diagnosis of Alzheimer's are varied and can change over time. You may find that you and your loved ones react in a similar manner, or you may have different responses. We all have different methods of coping with challenging information. Try to be aware of your reactions to the diagnosis and how they are affecting your ability to make necessary adjustments while continuing to live meaningfully. Life does not end when Alzheimer's is diagnosed.

Questions for Discussion

- How did you react to the diagnosis of Alzheimer's? Do you identify with any of the responses discussed in this chapter?
- Has your reaction to the diagnosis changed over time?
- If your loved ones or friends know about your diagnosis, how have they reacted? What kinds of reactions are helpful? Are there reactions that are hurtful or unhelpful?

Suggestions for Managing Your Reactions to the Diagnosis

- You have likely dealt with difficult news at other times in your life. Reflect on how you have managed or responded to other challenging news. Have your reactions helped or hindered your coping?
- Try to discuss your reaction to the diagnosis with a few trusted people. Talking about your reaction can help you process the news and makes others aware of how you are coping. If you are a private person or not willing or able to acknowledge the diagnosis, your loved ones may need their own support in coming to terms with your diagnosis.
- If you continue to react to the diagnosis of Alzheimer's with denial or significant anger, perhaps you would be more comfortable just trying to acknowledge that you have some memory loss. What you call the problem is less important than your ability to acknowledge that changes in your memory are beginning to impact your daily life.

Symptoms You Could Experience

This chapter provides an overview of common symptoms in early-stage Alzheimer's. Keep in mind that each person experiences Alzheimer's differently, and you may relate to some of these symptoms more than others. Many symptoms have a gradual onset or may vary in their significance or duration. Understanding symptoms is an essential part of learning about Alzheimer's for both you and your loved ones. We discuss specific ways to *manage* these symptoms in Part Three.

> *You have far more ability than you do disability. Focus on what you can do and don't lose sight of your strengths.*

Significant Memory Loss is the Most Common Symptom

Memory loss is the primary symptom of Alzheimer's disease. As we age, our memory functions become slower. It takes longer to learn something or to retrieve information from memory. One of the earliest symptoms of

Alzheimer's, however, is great difficulty learning and remembering *new* information. You may remember an event that occurred 30 years ago, but forget that you have a doctor's appointment today. This memory difficulty begins to affect daily organization and routine abilities. It is harder to keep up with appointments, maintain a checkbook, or cook a complex meal.

If you think of the brain as a huge filing cabinet, you are continually filing new information, storing it, and then retrieving it at a later time when needed. Memories can be stored across many regions of the brain, but the small area known as the hippocampus is primarily involved in receiving new information, temporarily storing it, and facilitating its move it into long-term filing. These memory processes happen through an elaborate set of electrical and chemical impulses and connections in the brain. The earliest effects of Alzheimer's begin in the hippocampus when abnormal protein deposits (plaques and tangles) begin to interrupt connections between brain cells. Although the hippocampus may receive new information temporarily, it can no longer retain the information and move it into longer-term memory. You may be able to understand new information at the time when it is presented to you, or be aware of something while it's happening, but later when you try to retrieve the information, it simply isn't there. In the book *The Majesty of Your Loving—A Couple's Journey Through Alzheimer's*, Harrison Hoblitzelle has Alzheimer's and says:

> "They're all here—the perceptions, ideas, and inspirations. They come in as before, but now they seem more fleeting. They're here, vivid, ready to express, but like a prairie dog, suddenly they disappear down a hole and they're gone… Now it's here. Now it's gone."[1]

Information and memories stored prior to the onset of Alzheimer's can still be retrieved because they are already in your brain's filing cabinet. Regions of the brain other than the hippocampus help to retrieve already-stored information. These regions may not be as affected until the later stages of the disease. So a memory filed away from childhood can be retrieved, while a new experience that never got into storage cannot.

You may wonder why you can remember certain current events or facts, but not others. You may forget what you watched on television the night before, yet a special recent occasion may be remembered with little effort. There is some evidence that information or experiences that have significant feelings associated with them—either strongly positive or negative feelings—may be processed and stored differently in the brain. These memories may receive an additional boost from the amygdala, a region of the brain involved with emotion. An emotionally powerful memory may be strengthened by the additional processing of the amygdala and, as a result, be more likely to get into the brain's storage system.

In general, however, memory is complex and variable, and it is common for people with Alzheimer's to have inconsistencies in their memory abilities.

It is Common to Lose or Misplace Things

Many people with Alzheimer's discuss their frustration with not being able to find things. You may place your wallet somewhere, but forget where you put it. Or you may start off looking for your wallet, go to where you think you left it, but once you get there, you forget what you were looking for. Harvey says, "I'll head outside to the tool shed to find a tool I need for a project and then, once I get there, I think to myself, 'Now what did I come out here for?'" You may begin to rely more on others to help you find things. One man writes:

> "I lose things. This is so common that I go to my wife and tell her what is missing and where I think I put it last. It isn't rare for her to say, 'Oh, that's over there.' She simply goes there and picks it up and hands it to me."[2]

Sometimes people with memory loss also put things in unusual places. Your wallet may end up in a kitchen cupboard or in some "special place" where you thought it would be safe. These special places can be hard to remember, and this contributes to difficulty in finding things. One person with Alzheimer's writes, "I often misplace things after thinking I have put them in a logical place. Then I can't remember my logic!"[3]

You Will Likely Repeat Yourself

A common symptom of memory loss is the tendency to repeat things you have already said or to ask the same question multiple times. Alzheimer's makes it difficult to remember conversations or to retain information. Bob describes the problem it poses for him and his wife. He says:

> "Unless we've talked about something for awhile, I will come back and ask Erika the same question over and over. I don't do it deliberately. It's just that each time it's like a new idea. And then I realize that it's not new and maybe we've talked about this more than once. She's patient. She doesn't say, 'Bob, you know you've already asked me that.' She just gives me the answer again. Maybe after three or four times I remember."[4]

Betty is also aware of how frustrating this dynamic can be for her husband:

> "Sometimes when I forget something, Kurt has to get hold of himself and not get all uptight about it. Obviously he's having to learn this over a period of time. It irritates me that he gets ticked off over something that I've forgotten and every once in awhile I blow up. I'm sorry about it, but I just forget things."[5]

Sometimes It's Hard to Find the Right Words

It is common for people with early-stage Alzheimer's to experience changes in verbal abilities. It may be harder for you to come up with the right word during conversation, or it may take longer for you to say something that would normally come easily. This symptom is called aphasia. Although anyone can experience word-finding problems occasionally, it is more common for people with Alzheimer's and can create frustrating moments in communication. Bill describes his word-finding difficulties:

> "For a while, I'll search for a word and I can see it walking away from me. It gets littler and littler. It always comes back, but at the wrong time. You can't be spontaneous."[6]

You may also mistakenly substitute one word for another during conversation. One person writes, "Often the word is close, but not as fitting as the one I had hoped to use before it disappeared."[7]

It is More Difficult to Complete Routine Tasks

Although you may know what you want to do, Alzheimer's can interfere with your ability to follow through. Many people have problems with staying organized. One man in a leadership position first became aware of these problems at work. He recalls, "I was looking for order…That's when I really knew I was having problems. I couldn't get organized…I just had a terrible desk and I couldn't seem to make it right."

Many activities that we take for granted, such as cooking, gardening, getting dressed, or enjoying a hobby, actually also involve a complex sequence of steps that require memory to complete. Alzheimer's makes it difficult to remember all of the steps of an activity or to get them in the right order. You may start off and get partway through a task and forget what you were trying to do or lose track of the next step. It may take you longer to do what you used to do with ease, and you may feel less motivated to try to accomplish tasks. Most people with Alzheimer's have to adjust their pace, slow down, and approach tasks one step at a time. Hank knows that these adjustments can be a challenge for both himself and his wife. He states:

"I say I can do it—I've done that hundreds of times. I don't want to admit defeat in doing anything I used to do. Having others take over because they are in a hurry makes it even harder for me to complete it and says to me I am useless. My support group facilitator said, 'Sometimes good enough is good enough.' That's what I need to teach my wife. I like that idea."

Some Things Might Look Different or be Hard to Recognize

If you rely on glasses or other corrective measures for vision, these will continue to be effective in helping you see clearly. However, you may find that although your vision is sharp, you don't always recognize what you see. This is called visual agnosia and is a particularly puzzling symptom of Alzheimer's. Bea describes her experience with this symptom, saying, "Sometimes what I'm looking for will be lying right in front of me and I won't see it. I don't always misplace things; they're right there, but I just don't recognize them."[8]

Anyone can have a similar experience occasionally, but the problem can be more frequent for people with Alzheimer's. Visual agnosia can affect the ability to identify familiar objects or sometimes even the ability to recognize people. People in the earlier stages of Alzheimer's have described moments when they didn't recognize a close family member or friend. Although these experiences can be frightening, they are usually temporary, might happen more often than people want to disclose, and do not necessarily represent severe disability.

Some people with Alzheimer's describe changes in their spatial and perceptual abilities. For example, colors may be hard to distinguish. A dark carpet may look like a hole in the floor or it may be hard to see a white plate on a cream-colored placemat. Sometimes it is difficult to judge distance or depth. You may reach for something and find that your hand lands inches away from the object, or the height of stairs or a sidewalk curb may be hard to determine and require greater caution when taking your steps.

You Might Get Disoriented in Familiar Places

Memory loss can make familiar places seem unfamiliar. You may be walking in your neighborhood and take a new route only to find that it is challenging to remember how to get home. Sometimes the disorientation passes quickly with a familiar landmark or other cue, or you may have difficulty finding your way one day and be perfectly oriented the next. Tom says:

> "You just don't know where you are for a moment…once in awhile I'll get to a place I don't know, and I've been there a hundred times before. And then it just snaps right in. Suddenly I'm where I'm supposed to be…just a feeling that I'm not here. Now I am here."[9]

Many people with Alzheimer's also have difficulty remembering directions to well-known destinations. It may also take a bit longer to orient yourself to new surroundings or to adjust to changes in your environment. While some people with early-stage Alzheimer's maintain a keen sense of direction, for others, disorientation can be a particularly frightening symptom. One man recalls, "I got separated from my wife for a few minutes in a shopping mall and it felt like I was lost for hours!"

Reading or Writing Could be More Challenging

Alzheimer's can impact both reading and writing. This is due to problems with memory and changes in visual abilities. Trouble with reading is called alexia, while problems with writing are known as agraphia. These symptoms can impact your enjoyment of certain activities. One man describes his challenges with reading: "The problem is if I'm reading a line and I get to the next line, I can't track the line. Reading isn't easy anymore. It's physically difficult." Others may find that their handwriting or typing abilities change, they have more trouble with spelling, or it becomes harder to put a thought into writing.

A Diminished Sense of Smell or Taste is Not Uncommon

Some decrease in smell is a normal part of aging, but Alzheimer's can make the loss more significant. The sense of smell is regulated by the olfactory bulb, which is located next to the hippocampus in the brain. The hippocampus, where we process memory, is usually the first area to be affected by Alzheimer's. Scientists think that due to its close proximity, the olfactory bulb may also be affected in the early stage of Alzheimer's. It may be harder for you to detect and identify smells. Reduced smell can also lead to reduced taste. Some people with Alzheimer's crave sweet or salty foods because these taste buds may continue to be sensitive for a longer period of time. Chronic sinus problems and smoking can also reduce one's sense of smell.

It is Common to Experience Mood Changes

People are capable of experiencing a wide range of feelings, and everyone can have changes in their mood throughout the day and throughout their lifetime. With Alzheimer's, mood changes can be temporary reactions to particular situations, or they may be more persistent due to changes in your brain. The onset of symptoms can be discouraging, frustrating, and frightening, and it is understandable to have a mix of emotional responses to these challenging events.

Alzheimer's can also make you more susceptible to intense emotions. It may be harder to control your feelings or they may be stronger than you have previously experienced. In contrast, some people have reduced emotional sensitivity. Some people may become more withdrawn, while others become more expressive. One person may be more fatigued while another experiences restlessness. Mood changes can affect your motivation to do things, your responses to daily events, and your outlook for the future. Shifts in mood can be challenging for both you and your loved ones, and it is helpful to talk with your doctor if changes in mood become extreme or disruptive to your daily life. (See Chapter 14 for a discussion of managing feelings.)

Feelings of Intimacy or Sexuality Can be Affected

Alzheimer's can affect both the physical and emotional aspects of intimacy and sexuality. You and your partner may experience shifts and changes in how you relate to one another as you both deal with the effects of Alzheimer's symptoms on your relationship. Increased feelings of stress, fatigue, depression, or irritability can reduce sex drive for both partners. Impotence is also common in men with Alzheimer's. Memory loss and other symptoms can result in diminished ability to be sensitive to a partner's needs or to previously enjoyed expressions of intimacy.

Some people with Alzheimer's can experience increased sex drive and may seek the reassurance of this form of intimacy to offset feelings of insecurity or loss. For others, sexual intimacy may reduce tension or provide comfort at a time of uncertainty or vulnerability. Regardless of the specific effects, most couples find that Alzheimer's does have an impact on the physical and emotional components of their sexual relationship, and you and your partner may each go through your own adjustments.

Many couples continue to exchange meaningful expressions of intimacy through a variety of physical or emotional means. One man says:

> "The closeness really extends to not only one thing. We are two people who were always close…Our closeness is intimacy. We go for walks, always hold hands. We talk."[10]

Others may struggle with more significant challenges and benefit from discussing these concerns with a physician or counselor. Although it may be difficult to talk about private matters, it is important to acknowledge any changes in intimacy or sexuality that are becoming disruptive to you and your care partner's relationship.

You Are More Than Your Symptoms

Symptoms of Alzheimer's vary considerably from person to person and can change over time. While it may be overwhelming to read about the possibilities, it is important to know that you are not at fault for any of these changes you may be experiencing. They are the result of a medical condition and, once identified, symptoms can often be managed through learning new methods of coping, finding support, or seeking medical attention. Sometimes so much focus is placed on how your symptoms may be affecting your life that it is easy to lose track of all of the ways in which they are *not* affecting it. You have far more ability than you do disability, and you have many capabilities. It is essential to focus on what you *can* do and not lose sight of your strengths. Diagnosed with Alzheimer's, retired psychologist Idel McLanathan writes in *Perspectives* newsletter:

"I know that my life's work as a family member, university professor, clinical psychologist, as a person in the world…my moments of self-satisfaction have been involved with times of helping others. I have sought to help my friends, my children, my students, my patients—and now, I hope, people I have yet to meet—realize that even when there are ways in which we are diminished, we must seek out that which is still ours to do—the things that give life meaning and that make us feel that 'we are worth our salt.' I cannot make flowers grow with much success. I cannot master difficult mathematic problems. I'm really not a notably admirable cook. The listing of my 'cannots' is not the subject. What is important is that I can feel that I accomplish something with my 'cans.' For example, what is making the present moment more positive for me is the hope that as you read these words, you will remember some of your 'of course I still can' abilities and that they lead you to greater appreciation of who you continue to be. Your desires and abilities—these are the important lists for you."[11]

Questions for Discussion

- Are you experiencing any of the symptoms described in this chapter? If so, which ones? How would you describe them?
- Are there other changes you are experiencing that may be due to Alzheimer's?
- Do you agree with your doctor or your loved ones about any symptoms you may be having? If not, why do you think others are suggesting that you have problems you may not be aware of?
- What are your strengths and abilities?

Suggestions for Understanding Possible Symptoms

- Anyone can occasionally experience the problems discussed in this chapter, but they happen more often when you have Alzheimer's. Recognize that you cannot always control how often or to what degree you experience symptoms, but you and others can learn effective ways of responding to them.
- Understand that each person with Alzheimer's is unique and it may or may not be helpful to compare your experience of symptoms with others' experiences.
- Make a list of your strengths. Ask your loved ones or another trusted person to help you expand your list. Although it is important to recognize Alzheimer's symptoms, you have many remaining abilities to draw on that deserve acknowledgment and attention.

Chapter Four

Talking with Others about Alzheimer's

If you have been diagnosed with Alzheimer's or a related disorder, you may have questions about how to share this news with others. Whom should I tell? Do I have to tell anyone? At what point should I start discussing this information? What should I say? How will people respond?

Although the news of Alzheimer's may be difficult, sometimes everyone feels relieved to have an explanation for the problem.

A Gradual Approach Can be Helpful

The first step in talking about your diagnosis with others is to come to terms with it yourself. This process of acceptance can be gradual. Some people with mild symptoms try to conceal their problems longer in order to maintain their self-image. One man says: "I don't care who knows or doesn't know. I don't try to hide it. Well, yes I do. I do try to hide it. You make a mistake or something and you try to hide it. I think it's natural. You don't want to appear to be less than you want to be. You want to appear as strong as you could be."[1] Each person's timing for telling others about the diagnosis varies. Bob says: "Why shouldn't I tell people about Alzheimer's? Why hide it? Otherwise they'll think, 'What is he doing?' I didn't tell people in the beginning. It wasn't until Alzheimer's became more prevalent—when I couldn't do things that I had done previously."[2]

It can be very challenging to accept the changes in your memory and other abilities. The process of acceptance may be less stressful, however, if you can rely on a few caring or understanding people to see you through the adjustments. Your family members may be the first ones you discuss your diagnosis with. You might also share this information with a few trusted friends or with community professionals who may be available through your local Alzheimer's organizations. You could be more comfortable talking about your diagnosis if you include discussions with others who are personally or professionally familiar with your symptoms.

Family and friends may also go through periods of denial by trying to ignore your problems or minimizing your concerns. Perhaps they attribute the changes to simply growing older, to stress, or to having a bad day now and then. But when the diagnosis is Alzheimer's, it is more likely that close family members or friends have noticed some of your symptoms and are concerned about you. Although the news of Alzheimer's may be difficult, sometimes everyone feels relieved to have an explanation for the problem. There is a medical reason for your memory loss or other symptoms. Discussing the diagnosis also means that you, your family, and your friends can make use of community or medical resources aimed at better understanding and treating your symptoms. Vaughn Collins writes:

> "My advice to others is to face the problem head-on and be open with family and friends. It helps me to have the love, support, and understanding from my immediate and extended family and close friends. My wife Rosella agrees that from the very beginning, we have not tried to keep the Alzheimer's experience secret."[3]

If you are a private person who is not comfortable with self-disclosure, perhaps you can give a family member or friend permission to discuss your diagnosis with others. It is important to respect your own needs for privacy while also considering the value of allowing selected people to know this information. Perhaps your spouse or family member has told someone about your Alzheimer's diagnosis without your consent. You may feel angry that you were not in charge of this decision, or maybe you are relieved that the decision was made for you. Try to understand that your family members also need support in this process, and they might be sharing the information in order to receive guidance or assistance.

Responses From Others

You may wonder how others will treat you if they know of your diagnosis. Perhaps you are concerned that others will back away from you or avoid you due to their own fears or discomfort. Although this may be true for some, others experience the opposite response. As public recognition of Alzheimer's and related disorders continues to grow, some people report that friends are supportive and do not treat them any differently from how they did before the diagnosis. Others describe how a kind stranger offered assistance with directions or provided other help once the condition was disclosed. Some people with early-stage Alzheimer's tell others about their diagnosis as a matter of safety and want others to know about their condition in case of an emergency. Lola reminds her ski club about her Alzheimer's and says, "If I don't come down off the mountain and get lost up on the slopes, I want someone to come looking for me!"[4] One man laughs as he discusses with his support group the caring but overprotective response of others on board a small cruise ship when he told them he had Alzheimer's: "They wouldn't let me out of their sight! I couldn't even go to the bathroom alone without someone trailing after me!"

You can't always predict how others will respond to your news, and sometimes you may just take a chance. Jean says:

"I've told my friends about Alzheimer's. They are very quiet. They don't know what to say. I don't know what to say. I think they understand because I'm telling them why it is so hard and the impact that the disease has. They listen. I don't expect them to respond any more than I could have responded two years ago before this happened to me. I don't expect more than to really have an opportunity to say what is going on and to express how I feel about it."[5]

Responses from some people may be helpful, while others are hurtful. Some people do not manage difficult information or circumstances effectively or sensitively. Others, however, will be respectful and caring when responding to your news. Consider letting them know what kinds of symptoms you are having and the most effective ways they can respond to them or help you deal with them. These conversations can put others at ease if they know that you are willing to acknowledge the problem and discuss it openly. After she was diagnosed with Alzheimer's, Maryalice Gordon wrote a letter to her friends in her church choir and gave them helpful tips for dealing with her memory loss. She writes:

"Please be patient with me if I look blankly when you tell me something that we just talked about yesterday or last week. Just repeat the information, and please without the 'I told you' or 'Don't you remember?' If we are planning something, please be sure that I write it down, or else give me a simple written note with instructions, date, time, and place. If I can see it, I can do it. If I can't see it, it doesn't exist! I may know your name now, but may not be able to recall it later. Nametags help. Please don't ignore me; I'm still here! Please don't be afraid to ask me questions. Sometimes I even know the answer!"[6]

Talking About Alzheimer's to Increase Public Awareness

Some people with Alzheimer's tell others about their diagnosis as a means of educating the public and decreasing stigma. Public awareness of Alzheimer's grows when people are willing to be open about their condition. Indeed, more recently a growing number of people with early-stage Alzheimer's are being profiled in news stories, speaking at conferences, and doing Alzheimer's advocacy work in their communities (see Chapter 18). These efforts can help to broaden awareness that people with Alzheimer's are able to learn ways to cope with challenging symptoms, contribute to their communities, and lead meaningful and satisfying lives. Diagnosed at age 52, Grace believes it is important for the public to be aware of the many faces of Alzheimer's and that it's no laughing matter. She remarks:

> "I tell everybody! It's nothing to be ashamed of. People need to know that we're just like them. The other day, I was in a store and I was in line to buy my dress. The cashier was making mistakes and joking, 'Oh no, I must have Alzheimer's!' When I got up to the register, I looked at her and I said, 'I do have Alzheimer's.' I think she was pretty embarrassed that she had joked about it."[7]

Increased public awareness can break down stereotypes and foster greater sensitivity to the experiences and needs of people with Alzheimer's. Those who are willing to be a public voice can also be powerful spokespersons in helping to advance progress in the development of research and valuable community-based programs.

Telling Others in Your Workplace About Alzheimer's

If you are still working, you may face sensitive decisions about when and how to discuss Alzheimer's in your workplace. While some people continue to work for as long as possible in the early stages of Alzheimer's, most find that memory loss and other symptoms begin to affect work performance. It may be stressful to try to fulfill routine work tasks, and you need to decide when to discuss your diagnosis with your employer. It is important to discuss with your doctor whether your symptoms could interfere with your ability to perform your job duties or with the safety or well-being of others who might rely on you.

If you work in a company or organization with a human resources or benefits department, you may want to start your discussion with someone there who can make you aware of your rights, including any work modifications, disability plans, or retirement benefits that you are entitled to. It is usually better to be up front about your diagnosis and secure any benefits that are available through your workplace rather than to wait too long and lose your job due to work performance problems. Depending on your job responsibilities, your employer may be able to make some modifications that allow you to continue working for as long as possible until symptoms interfere. If you are self-employed, you may need to rely on your doctor, family, or a close friend to help you accurately assess your ability to continue in your job.

Sometimes others are aware of problems or observe changes in your work performance even when you may think you are functioning well. Try to find a few trusted people to confide in about your diagnosis so you can review your circumstances with them. It can be helpful to obtain a written explanation of your employment benefits that you can share with a loved one or advocate who may be helping you work through these job-related decisions. As a growing number of people stay in the workforce into more advanced age, dealing with the impact of early-stage Alzheimer's or related disorders in the workplace will likely become more common.

Each person may manage decisions about disclosing the diagnosis of Alzheimer's to others differently. Eventually, however, others will become aware of your symptoms, and it is usually better to take charge of telling others rather than to avoid the process indefinitely. Although some people might shy away when they hear the word "Alzheimer's," you may also make new friends as a result of the discussion. Who knows? You may be talking with someone who has just been diagnosed, too!

Questions for Discussion

- Who should know about your diagnosis? Are there people you don't want to tell? Why?
- What concerns do you have about possible responses from others? How might you deal with varied responses?
- What are the possible benefits of telling others about Alzheimer's?

Suggestions for Discussing Your Diagnosis with Others

- Make a list of the people who should be informed of your diagnosis. This may include family, close friends, or an employer.
- Discuss with your care partner any differences of opinion about whom and when to tell. If there is a conflict, try to understand each other's perspective. How would each of you feel if you were in the other's position? Are you concerned about your privacy or about how others will respond? Would you feel differently about telling others if the diagnosis was a different medical problem? Try to find a compromise so that the needs of both you and your loved ones are respected.
- Write a letter to family and friends to tell them about the diagnosis. This lifts the burden of having to repeat the news over again to each person.
- Let others know what you need from them or what might be helpful in response to your diagnosis. Try to advise them on ways they can better understand and respond to your memory loss or other symptoms.
- Obtain pamphlets from your regional Alzheimer's organizations to give to those who want or need more information. Refer family and friends to these organizations for further information.

Chapter Five

Taking Care of Family Relationships

There are few things more central to our lives than family relationships. Your family may be large or small. You may have close connections with one another, or perhaps your relationships are more distant or challenging and vary between different family members. Regardless of your family makeup and dynamics, memory loss and other symptoms of Alzheimer's can result in gradual shifts and changes in these relationships. For many people with Alzheimer's, common issues arise as they discuss their feelings and concerns about the effects of symptoms on the family. As you read this chapter, think about which themes you identify with and how you are dealing with them in your own family.

> *"At first I wanted to protect my family. But I decided that it is more important to be honest with family right from the beginning."*

Family Denial or Confusion

The early stages of Alzheimer's can be very confusing for family members and can create conflict in relationships. The day-to-day variability in your symptoms can lead family members to question the accuracy of the diagnosis or the reality of the problem. It may be hard to understand why you remember some things but not others and why some tasks are easy to accomplish while others have become challenging. Family members who have less contact with you may not see the changes in you as clearly as those who are with you more often. These early-stage issues can result in family members having conflicting impressions of the significance of your symptoms, with some members minimizing the problems or accusing others of exaggerating them.

Perhaps you, too, want to minimize the significance of your symptoms or try to cover them up. This can make matters even more confusing for everyone. A participant of a support group in Ontario, Canada, says:

> "I have always wanted to tell my family members about how hard this diagnosis is for me and the problems that go along with it. I have not told them because I want to keep a positive attitude and I need them to help me. At first I wanted to protect my family from knowing what may happen to me as this disease progresses, because I didn't want them to be scared or feel bad, but I decided that it is more important to be honest with family right from the beginning."[1]

It is very common in the early stages of Alzheimer's for you and your family members to experience many different stages of awareness and acceptance and to not always be in agreement. If you have always been a private person, or if honest and open discussion is difficult, you may find it helpful to seek assistance from an Alzheimer's specialist who can facilitate a family meeting to discuss these sensitive issues.

Making Adjustments to Symptoms

Although some people with Alzheimer's live alone, most have contact with a primary support person such as a spouse, son, daughter, other relative, or close friend. You may be concerned about the impact of symptoms on these loved ones, and each family member or friend might have to make some adjustments. Everyone has to learn about the unpredictable and often frustrating experience of memory loss. This can take time, and not everyone adjusts at the same rate. As one man with Alzheimer's recently told his social worker, "Will you please remind my wife not to forget that I forget?"

Although you may realize that your loved ones have assumed more responsibilities since the onset of your symptoms, some people with Alzheimer's are less aware that their condition has had an impact on others. It can be helpful to have a discussion with family members about any adjustments that all of you are making. Try to work together to determine what would lessen any stress. A support group or educational class can be a valuable resource for you and your family to help all of you better understand your symptoms. One woman describes the benefit of a support group in her husband's acceptance process:

> "My husband wanted me to shape up. He didn't want to think I had Alzheimer's. He was scared. He has stopped asking me, 'Don't you remember?' and I am so proud of him."

It can be helpful to talk with others who are experiencing similar circumstances, and the camaraderie and sharing in such programs can help to ease the adjustment process. (See Chapter 15 for a discussion of support groups.)

Expect Some Shifts in Responsibilities and Roles

Because of Alzheimer's symptoms, you will gradually need more assistance from others. This may result in changes in relationship roles for you and your loved ones. Often this creates considerable adjustments that are best made gradually when possible. One woman reflects on her relationship with her husband:

We express our caring and appreciation of each other more now and don't take that for granted."

Relationships with Children and Adolescents

If you developed Alzheimer's at a younger age, you may have your own young children still at home (see Chapter 6). More likely, you have grandchildren or great-grandchildren now, or you have relationships with other young people in your extended family or community. Although most of the educational and support services for families facing Alzheimer's are directed to adults, these children or adolescents in your life may also be affected by your condition and have their own concerns.

Young people often notice memory changes in their family member or elderly friend, but may be cautious to ask about the problems or to discuss them. Encourage young people to ask you any questions they have about Alzheimer's. Children can be especially direct, so be prepared for candid questions. They may need help to better understand your memory loss or other symptoms and to learn ways of coping with and responding to the changes you are experiencing.

Family members of all ages can support one another in developing positive responses to challenges. Some adolescents who take on new responsibilities in helping a loved one with Alzheimer's develop a closer bond with that loved one and feel good about being needed and valued. Other young people, however, may feel burdened by any caregiving responsibilities or resentful that they are receiving less attention due to the needs of the family member with Alzheimer's. Children may not know how to explain their family member's symptoms to their peers and may struggle to find their own support.

Just as young people may differ in their responses to the person with Alzheimer's, people with Alzheimer's also differ in their responses to young people. You may feel more easily overwhelmed with the onset of memory problems, and the energy of youth may be tiring or irritating. Or, you may find that young people are a highlight in your life and value the time you spend with them. One woman says:

"I really enjoy being with my grandkids because they are always changing and each day is like a new discovery for them and for me. I like to read to them. They love it. They are pretty little, so their books have large print and that's a lot easier for me to read these days."

Your family relationships will undergo shifts and changes as you all adapt to the effects of Alzheimer's on your lives. Although there will be challenges and adjustments, you can work now to set a solid foundation for teamwork and open communication. Use this time to build on your strengths and seek help as necessary to resolve significant differences so you can move forward together.

Questions for Discussion

- Is everyone in your family aware of your diagnosis? How are they responding or adjusting to your symptoms?
- Are there role changes within your family relationships? If so, what are they and how do you feel about them?
- Has your family faced other challenges together in the past? What are your family's strengths and weaknesses when coping with challenges?
- Do you have children or adolescents in your life? How are they responding?

Suggestions for Strengthening Family Relationships

- Sometimes family relationships begin to revolve around responsibilities and obligations, and family members lose sight of the value of recreational time. Have fun together! Plan enjoyable activities or trips to do together.
- If you have limited or no family support, a few key friends or professionals from community agencies can help to build the support needed now and in the future (see Chapter 13 for more on living alone with Alzheimer's).

- If you are having conflict or difficulty communicating with family members, call your local Alzheimer's organizations for a referral to a counselor who can help you and your loved ones discuss concerns.
- Make sure that children or adolescents have the information they need about Alzheimer's. If young people reach out to you, think of ways they might be able to assist you, such as running an errand or making you a cup of tea. Show your appreciation so that they feel valued and useful.
- Explore whether there are educational programs available in your community for families facing early-stage Alzheimer's or a related disorder, including specialized programs for children and adolescents.

Chapter Six

The Unique Concerns of Young-Onset Alzheimer's Families

When most people think of Alzheimer's or a related disorder, they assume it is affecting someone who is elderly. Although age is the greatest risk factor for Alzheimer's, in recent years, scientists and the public have become increasingly aware of people who develop Alzheimer's or a related disorder before age 65. These individuals range in age from their late 20s to their early 60s and have what is termed "early-onset" or "young-onset" Alzheimer's.

> *"I always expected to get ill or have Alzheimer's when I got older, not now when I'm in my 30s."*

"I'm Too Young To Have Alzheimer's!"

If you have young-onset Alzheimer's, you have the same condition as those diagnosed at an older age, and your symptoms and rate of change will be just as varied. Although you may hear that people with young-onset Alzheimer's have a more rapid progression in their symptoms, this is not necessarily so, and research does not consistently support this prevailing belief. Younger individuals and families do, however, experience unique challenges. For many, finances are a concern. You may be at the peak of your career and earning the money necessary for retirement or other expenses. The onset of disability requires different financial and long-term planning. If you are in the middle of raising a family with dependent children or young adults still at home or in college, your children will have their own needs that could require attention and support. Since many social and support programs for persons with Alzheimer's are primarily directed to older participants, it may be more challenging for you and your family to find a peer group or services and programs geared to younger families facing Alzheimer's. Although all of these challenges are significant, there is now much more attention being given to young-onset families and it is possible to build a community and find assistance as needed. The first step is making sure that you get a thorough evaluation and have the attention of a good healthcare provider.

Understanding Rare Genetic Factors

Some rare cases of young-onset Alzheimer's are the result of certain gene mutations (located on chromosomes 1, 14, and 21) that are passed down through families. A parent with young-onset Alzheimer's caused by one of these genetic mutations has a 50 percent chance of passing the gene on to his or her children. If a child inherits the gene from the parent, that child is certain to develop Alzheimer's, usually at about the same young age that the parent developed the disease. Multiple members of a family can be affected. In these families, individuals who do not yet have symptoms can be tested to see if they carry the gene. This is a profoundly significant decision, as it can determine with relative certainly the likelihood of developing this form of familial Alzheimer's. Some people want this information as a means of planning for their future; others would rather not know and would prefer to let time tell.

When doctors do a comprehensive evaluation of memory loss or other symptoms in a young person with a strong family history of young-onset Alzheimer's, they often seek testing for these genetic mutations to confirm a diagnosis. Researchers are also interested in these young-onset families and may want genetic testing in order to gain better understanding of how these genes work. Regardless, comprehensive counseling and informed consent must always accompany any genetic testing. Consuelo, who was tested for a familial gene, points out that it's important not to be pressured to get genetic testing:

> "It should be you who wants to do it. You have to make sure in advance that you know what you're getting into. You have to consider all the pros and cons of knowing the results, and see if you think you can handle them before being tested. Choose the decision that you want, not what someone else wants. And even if you're tested, you don't have to get the results. You can do it just to benefit science."[1]

It is important to understand that most cases of young-onset Alzheimer's are not due to identified genes, and scientists are not always certain why symptoms begin in someone at an earlier age.

Responding to Disbelief

Many young-onset individuals describe difficulty in getting their symptoms evaluated by a doctor. Symptoms may be attributed to mid-life crisis, depression, changes from menopause, or stress. One woman diagnosed with Alzheimer's in her early 60s states:

> "People tend not to believe that I have anything wrong because I look and sound so healthy. One of my major stresses was getting a doctor to believe that it's more than stress, depression, or burnout."[2]

If you are reading this book, chances are that your doctor has ruled out other possible causes of your symptoms and made a diagnosis of Alzheimer's or a related dementia. If not, it is important that you see a neurologist (a doctor who specializes in the brain and nervous system) for a complete evaluation of your symptoms (see Chapter 1). If you have been thoroughly evaluated and diagnosed, let your family and friends know that it's time to acknowledge the problem and that you need their support in coming to terms with the diagnosis.

Facing Early Retirement and Financial Challenges

Some people with mild symptoms of Alzheimer's are able to continue working at their jobs for a limited period of time. If you are employed, consider your work responsibilities and the impact that your symptoms may have on your work performance. Depending on your employment responsibilities, the onset of memory loss and other symptoms could make it difficult to continue performing your job. Sometimes co-workers notice problems with work performance. One man says:

> "I did not sense I was having difficulty and my wife didn't either. Some people I worked with started noticing I did things that weren't quite what they thought I would normally do. They went to a supervisor. Fortunately, she took the path of calling me in and telling me what she had heard. It was a blow."[3]

It may be possible to have modifications made in your job that allow you to stay in it longer, but this requires that you disclose your diagnosis to your employer or to a counselor in the human resources department. The Americans with Disabilities Act includes laws that protect the rights of persons with disabilities in the workplace, and it will be important to learn how these laws may apply to you. Your roles or responsibilities could be adjusted as needed for a limited period of time so you can stay in the workforce for as long as possible.

Depending on your job or profession, it could be challenging to continue working, and the difficulty of trying to manage work responsibilities may create added stress. Young-onset Alzheimer's occurs during the years when many people are trying to earn the income necessary for a comfortable retirement, and you may have significant concerns about the financial and social impact of early retirement. One young-onset person says:

> "There is a unique problem for those of us who are working and have been informed we are no longer able to perform our duties. We're not financially prepared to retire, and it is difficult to qualify for various kinds of insurance. I applied for Social Security Disability only to be told I was ineligible."[4]

Applications for disability can be complex and benefits are based on your work history, the documentation of your symptoms and diagnosis, and the distribution of any other benefits you may be receiving. Sometimes it is necessary to appeal a decision if you think you are eligible for benefits but are denied.

In February 2010, the Social Security Administration added young-onset Alzheimer's and other young-onset dementias to the list of conditions under its Compassionate Allowance Initiative so that disability applications from these individuals can be expedited and processed with greater ease and priority. This is hopeful progress in ensuring that young-onset individuals are afforded any benefits that they are entitled to as soon as possible and with limited obstacles.

Legal and financial planning is essential to address the adjustments and changes in income and expenses brought on by disability. It becomes particularly important with young-onset disability, and applying for benefits is indeed confusing. (See Chapter 26 for information about legal and financial planning.) If you lose your job, you may also be at risk of losing healthcare benefits, and you should discuss healthcare options with your employer. Young-onset persons who are disabled for two years or more are eligible for Medicare, and Alzheimer's advocates are currently appealing Congress to reduce the time between diagnosis and Medicare eligibility. If you have limited income, you may be eligible for the federal Medicaid program. Your local Alzheimer's organization should be able to connect you with a social worker or other disability rights advocate who can help determine your eligibility for benefits.

If You Have Children Living at Home

In many families with young-onset Alzheimer's, it is not uncommon to find children or adolescents still living in the home. Children may experience many different feelings as they try to cope with the changes in their affected parent. They may need care from the parent at the same time that the affected parent is starting to need more assistance. There may be added stressors placed on young family members as they try to juggle the responsibilities of both school and home. Sometimes these challenges can draw a family closer, but there may also be awkward or difficult times when roles are changing and family members (including the person with Alzheimer's) have to make significant adjustments. Bill, diagnosed at age 54, says, "My sons are dealing with this very well. They're good kids." However, he adds, "They used to learn from me, and now I have to learn from them. I don't really like it. I feel like it's topsy-turvy, but that's the way it has to be."[5]

If you have children at home, it is important to consider their age and stage of development, as this will affect both their emotional and practical needs. Children of all ages may require your parenting in ways that can become challenging. If you are responsible for their meal preparation, organizing their activities, helping with homework, and other responsibilities, these tasks may become more difficult to manage and you may need to develop new strategies for staying involved in these responsibilities. There are still, however, many ways to be an active and involved parent. One woman diagnosed in her early 50s writes:

> "It seems so unfair for my kids to have to shoulder this new lifestyle. But deep in my heart, I know I still have precious time

to listen to them and be a present figure in their lives…I know that now is the time to teach them about life and to support them, and help them grow strong with compassionate hearts. In that, I find a will to fight this thing as long as I can."[6]

Children could have emotional responses to your symptoms that depend somewhat on their age and their pre-existing temperament. Elementary school children may be confused or frightened by the changes in your abilities and will need reassurance, comfort, and a basic understanding of your Alzheimer's symptoms. Older adolescents and teenagers may need more detailed information about your diagnosis, or in contrast, may be so absorbed in their own life issues that they may not be as sensitive to your own. Some children are candid about a parent's changing abilities and benefit from direct communication. Others may internalize their feelings or thoughts and be reluctant to talk. Pay close attention to any change in academic performance, social relationships, or daily routines in your children that may indicate stress or difficulty coping. School counselors or Alzheimer's specialists can be helpful resources for support as needed.

Finding Peers and Meaningful Activity

If you are younger with Alzheimer's, it can be difficult to find social activity and support because your spouse or friends may still be working during the daytime or busy raising a family. If you derived satisfaction and social stimulation from work, it is important to find ways to maintain or build social interactions. For some, meeting others with Alzheimer's can begin to open up new relationships. Since the majority of people with Alzheimer's are over age 65, you may be in support groups or other programs with people up to 40 years your senior, but people with Alzheimer's often find that they share common symptoms, concerns, coping strategies, and opportunities to support one another regardless of age. Bill recalls the first early-stage support group meeting that he and his wife attended:

"When the first day came, I was a bit nervous, but I looked forward to meeting new friends that I could relate to. When we first glanced at the group, I thought we were in the wrong room because everyone else was at least 10 or 20 years older than us. But that distinction began to melt away when we found that we were all in the same boat and in that sense, all the same age."[7]

It is important to give any available early-stage support or activity programs a try, because you may find that there are other younger people with Alzheimer's or a related disorder in your community, and rewarding friendships can grow from shared empathy and experiences.

Persons with young-onset Alzheimer's are often physically healthy with considerable energy, and it can be challenging to find ways to channel that energy. Community-based activities for people with Alzheimer's may be more accommodating to the social and physical norms of an older population. Some communities are beginning to develop special programs for young-onset families in an attempt to build social connections and decrease potential feelings of isolation. Since many younger families are accustomed to using computers, an international email network has been established for online communication and sharing as well as a newsletter for young-onset individuals and families. One person says:

"I don't do very well on the phone because I can't remember long conversations, so I prefer email. So that got to be my support group. I have 'met' early-onset people from all around the country and we kind of made our own little support group."[8]

More information about this network is available at the Oklahoma/Arkansas Chapter of the Alzheimer's Association at 918-481-7741 or www.alz.org/alzokar.

Some people feel an added sense of urgency to capitalize on their health and physical energy for as long as possible. Thirty-four-year-old Consuelo says:

"I don't know if it's harder at my age than it would be if I were 70. Maybe it would be the same. But I always expected to get ill or have Alzheimer's when I got older, not now when I'm in my 30s. It does make me want to do things now, like traveling, that I might have postponed until later years. I want to see London and Paris."[9]

Others channel their energy into meaningful advocacy work to raise money for Alzheimer's research and services and to increase public awareness (see Chapter 18). Chuck Jackson has a genetic, familial form of Alzheimer's that has resulted in his early-onset symptoms. As a member of the baby-boom generation, he feels it is important to educate the public and Congress about the many faces of Alzheimer's and the unique concerns of younger people. He writes about his trip to Washington, D.C. for the Alzheimer's Association annual advocacy days:

"As our meetings progressed for the three days of training, more and more persons with dementia arrived. I found myself talking to people my own age; some younger, some older, but people with early-onset Alzheimer's. We compared notes on drugs, symptoms, and emotions dealing with the disease. Many of them told me that they came just to hear me speak on early-onset issues. They were thrilled that we were being acknowledged and listened to. It is a marvelous thing to see folks from all over the nation gathering to change the face of Alzheimer's disease."[10]

As the baby-boom generation ages, the numbers of people with young-onset Alzheimer's are likely to increase, and there have already been important strides made around the world to draw attention to their particular challenges. Although people diagnosed younger in life often experience unique concerns, there are also many shared experiences among people with Alzheimer's, regardless of age. It is important to reach out and find both professionals and peers who will help you navigate this journey and make the most of the years ahead.

Questions for Discussion

- Did you have difficulty obtaining a diagnosis? Do you feel you have a good relationship with your healthcare team now?
- Do you have young children at home? If so, how have they responded to your symptoms? If you have older children, how are they managing?
- If you are no longer able to work, are there other ways you would like to try to channel your energy?
- Have you met others with Alzheimer's? Has your age posed any barrier to building relationships?

Suggestions for Young-Onset Families

- If you must retire from work early, seek immediate legal or estate planning advice so you can plan effectively for the future.
- Contact your local Alzheimer's organizations to see if they are aware of young-onset programs or other young-onset families in your community so you can be introduced to others. Make use of online networks to connect with others with young-onset symptoms.
- If you have difficulty finding other young families facing Alzheimer's, consider contacting other societies for conditions such as Multiple Sclerosis, Huntington's disease, Frontotemporal Dementia, or Parkinson's disease. These neurological conditions often affect individuals at a younger age and you may have common concerns.
- Obtain age-appropriate educational information for children through your local Alzheimer's organizations. Let school counselors or teachers know about your diagnosis so they can be sensitive to your child's needs or concerns in the classroom.
- You and your family members may benefit from counseling or professional guidance to help with adjustments and to develop coping skills together.

Chapter Seven

Maintaining Friendships and Creating New Ones

For most people, relationships with friends and a social community are a meaningful part of daily life. Positive relations with others are important in maintaining your social, functional, and communication abilities. Although Alzheimer's does not change the significance of these relationships, you may be concerned about the impact of Alzheimer's on your friendships. It could be more challenging to participate in hobbies and activities you previously enjoyed with your friends, or changes in language and communication abilities may mean that conversations take more effort. Perhaps you no longer drive, so transportation to activities is more complicated. These changes can lead to a risk of social isolation, and it is important to continue to interact with others in whatever way feels most comfortable.

> *Meeting new friends can be an unexpected positive outcome of having Alzheimer's.*

Who Are Your Friends?

Each person has a unique community of friends. You may have a large network of friends whom you have met through specific interests, a shared faith, or common experiences. Perhaps you have friendships that span many years of building a history together and seeing one another through challenging times. These friendships likely involve greater communication, disclosure, and trust. If you have moved recently for retirement or to live closer to family, you may have left a community of friends behind and not yet established a new one. While long-standing and long-distance friendships can be comforting, you may also need new friends to help form your community during this time.

Perhaps you have been a less socially active person, are more solitary, and have a smaller group of friends. Maybe you have relied on a spouse or partner to maintain the social connections in the relationship and are less comfortable initiating friendships on your own. If you have been more reserved, it is important to understand that there may be new people coming into your life. Few people with Alzheimer's or their care partners can manage without the eventual assistance or support of others, and you may find that there are satisfactions and benefits from forming relationships at this time.

With the onset of Alzheimer's, it can be helpful to take stock of your friendships and your community. Who are your friends, and how satisfied are you with these relationships? You may have different social needs than your care partner, and this is also important to take into consideration. If you live alone, being aware of your community or beginning to establish one is essential (see Chapter 13).

What Your Friends Need to Know

At some point, you need to decide what your friends should know about your diagnosis and symptoms. You might talk to some friends right away, but choose to remain private with others. You may feel relieved to get the matter out in the open, or you may be reluctant to reveal too much. Your own experience with symptoms will also influence what you share with others. If you are often bothered by your memory loss or are self-conscious about other symptoms, telling friends about your experiences can be a helpful way for them to gain understanding into Alzheimer's and be more sensitive in their relationship with you. One woman says, "My friends don't really treat me much differently since I developed Alzheimer's. I've told them about my condition, so if I do something goofy, I've got a good excuse!"[1]

When Friends Offer Their Help or Support

If you tell your friends about Alzheimer's, they may want to offer help or support, but not know how. You and your care partner will benefit from thinking about specific ways people can continue to stay involved in your life. Perhaps that means that one friend goes out to lunch with you once a month while another friend makes sure you continue to get to your golf game, book club, or other hobby you enjoy together. Maybe one friend can be counted on for emotional support during the tough times, while another friend is better at distracting you from your feelings with a fun activity.

When people offer their support, they need to know what is helpful to you. You or your care partner might hope that close friends can read your mind and know what you need, but most people need guidance about how they can be helpful during this challenging time. Try to examine your expectations of your friends and work toward a realistic and mutual understanding of how to maintain these meaningful relationships.

If Your Friends Are No Longer Friendly

Friends do not always come through in the ways we might hope. Some friends might back away because they are uncomfortable with your symptoms, or perhaps they are trying to manage their own challenges and have limited energy. Others may be friendships based on a shared hobby or activity with you, and if you are no longer able to participate, the friendship dissolves. It can be hurtful to experience losses in relationships, but it is important to take an honest look at these friendships, adjust your expectations, and let go of the relationship if necessary. Ron speaks about painful challenges with some of his friendships in the Canadian video *I Have Alzheimer's Disease*. He says:

"They are staying away from me because it's too awkward…I now think that I'm going to buy into the theory that it's not my fault…I'm going to tell it like it is and if they don't come back, they don't come back. We'll just find out who's on my team."[2]

When you acknowledge that some friendships are lost, you are more able to move on and open the door to new possibilities. Some people find that meeting new friends is an unexpected positive outcome from having Alzheimer's. You may form new bonds with others through Alzheimer's-related support groups or other activities and develop friendships based on shared concerns and the ease of camaraderie with others who understand your feelings and experiences.

Creating Connections with Others

The need for friendship and the extent of one's community varies greatly from person to person. You may be satisfied with one or two close friends, or you may have always valued a larger network of relationships. Each person is unique, but it is important for your physical and mental health that you not become isolated from others as a result of Alzheimer's. Continued social interaction also helps to stimulate your language and other thinking abilities and is an important part of maintaining well-being. It is not uncommon to hear stories from people with Alzheimer's and their care partners about the new friends they have made as a result of the diagnosis. There is much research that confirms the value of social support during stressful times, and it can be very helpful to form friendships with people who share similar concerns or who help you to carry on with valued routines or activities in life.

Shimon Camiel retired from his profession in public health, but continues to apply the principles of his profession to his current concerns about living with Alzheimer's. He writes in *Perspectives* newsletter:

"I have a feeling of sadness for people who are isolated. You need warmth, especially initially, when you find out you have this disease. I had so many people around me when I was diagnosed. That was my comfort and my community. I think that's why I landed on my feet. For a half a year or so, I was feeling sorry for myself, but now I'm having a great time. I guess there are people hiding in a closet who never get out, but in general people need to touch people and to surround each other and feel connected, even if you don't have Alzheimer's… I don't want community to be just a lucky occurrence—it's part of what decency is. We need that so much. We need to give some time to thinking about that and how to make that happen."[3]

A growing number of communities have developed special programs or educational events that bring families facing early-stage Alzheimer's together for support. Other communities or rural regions may have more limited opportunities. If there are no specialized programs in your community, call your local chapter of the Alzheimer's Association or other regional Alzheimer's organization to see if there are ways to meet other families in your area who are living with Alzheimer's. Your social life and sense of community may undergo shifts and changes, but being open-minded to the benefits of maintaining friendships and creating new ones can open the door for positive experiences and potentially rewarding relationships.

Questions for Discussion

- Who are your friends? Are you satisfied with the number and kinds of friendships that you have?
- What have you told your friends about Alzheimer's? How have they responded?
- Have any of your friendships changed as a result of your having Alzheimer's? If so, how?
- Do you think it would be helpful to form new friendships with others who have Alzheimer's? Why or why not?

Suggestions For Maintaining and Making Friendships

- Write a list of your friends or your support team. Include family as well as trusted friends or professionals. Are you satisfied with the list?
- If you are cautious about sharing the news of your diagnosis with others, consider starting with one or two of your closest friends. If you are uncomfortable having this discussion in person or your friends are long-distance, consider writing a letter to them.
- Think of the activities you like to do. Are they solitary or do they involve others? Although some people are less social than others, make sure that some of your daily activities include socialization with others.
- Explore social programs that might be available to you in your community through the Alzheimer's Association or other related organizations. If there are no programs for people with early-stage Alzheimer's, ask that one be started!

Chapter Eight

Strategies for Effective Communication with Friends and Family

Most people rely on verbal communication as a primary form of expression. For many people with Alzheimer's, changes in their language and speaking abilities are some of the first recognizable symptoms. These challenges with communication are generally referred to as aphasia. This chapter addresses some of the most common experiences with aphasia and discuss effective strategies for improving communication.

> *It is important to continue participating in conversations and for others to include you.*

"I Forgot What I Was Going to Say!"

Memory loss is the primary symptom of Alzheimer's, and it can interfere with communication. Many people describe losing their train of thought mid-sentence or forgetting what they wanted to say during a conversation. This process can become very frustrating and complex. Dick Barlow writes:

> "The main problem is that I start to say something, and suddenly I don't know what I'm trying to say. I don't know how to say it, and whatever I was trying to say is gone. The subject, the means of communication, the words I'm about to use next, they disappear. It's outrageously exasperating! Just murderous! Maybe the next day I'll remember what I wanted to say. And then I have to be careful because if I switch over to the thought that I just now remembered and start talking about it, I am highly likely to lose track of any other conversation we might presently be having. I have to quickly decide whether to switch and talk about yesterday's thought because it may not last long."[1]

Many people can get back on track in their conversation with some gentle prompting. One man tells his support group:

> "Sometimes I'll start a sentence and forget what it is I was going to say halfway through. But if someone prompts me by repeating the part of the sentence I've already said, then often I can pick up my train of thought and finish the sentence."

Others may be frustrated by premature attempts from others to help. You may feel pressured if you sense someone else's impatience with your communication, and pressure can make your problem worse. Yvonne states:

> "My husband was finishing my words, finishing my thoughts. I took him aside privately and said it wasn't helping. I said, 'I know you are trying to help, but it's just making me mad. If I stumble around, let me.' Unless you tell a person, 'This is not helping me,' they don't know…You have to say how you feel."[2]

Friends and family often struggle with knowing when to step back and let you find your train of thought or when to step in and try to assist. Others may not always have the right clue to get you back on track, but most likely their attempts to help are sincere. They are trying their best to help, and your gentle feedback can be constructive in guiding their attempts.

It is important to continue participating in conversation and for others to include you. The more you continue to communicate, the better others can become at understanding your train of thought, your stumbling blocks, and the strategies that work best in helping you express yourself.

Sometimes the Words Just Disappear

Difficulty with finding words is common for people with Alzheimer's and is called *anomia.* Some describe the problem as a word being "on the tip of my tongue," or like a sudden empty gap that interrupts the flow of thought. You may have a thought in your head and begin to express it, but find that you get stuck partway through and can't find a necessary word. Or, you think you are about to say a certain word but when you go to speak, something totally different comes out! This can be quite a surprise, and scientists call these incidents *paraphasic errors.* In his book *Partial View*, Cary Henderson describes his experience with anomia:

> "The words get tangled very easily, and I get frustrated when I can't think of a word. Every time I converse with somebody, there's always some word I can't remember. I really cuss when I can't remember a word."[3]

Some people find that by the time they get the word out, it is difficult to remember their train of thought to complete their sentence. A woman confides to friends in an early-stage Alzheimer's social club, saying, "I lose one word and then I can't come up with the rest of the sentence. I just stop talking and people think something is really wrong with me!"[4] Kay is more outspoken about her communication lapses and says with a chuckle, "I admit it—I've just had a senior moment!"

If you experience anomia, try to simplify what you want to say and allow more time to express yourself. When you are rushed, the problem worsens. If you cannot think of a word, try to find another substitute instead of fighting the problem, or ask for help from the person with whom you are speaking. It is sometimes surprising how someone else may be able to guess what you are trying to say and save you a lot of effort! One woman has developed the following effective strategy with her adult children:

> "When in public, I would like my children to step in and help me with what I am trying to communicate. I give my children a look. We joke about it being a 'mother's look'—you know the look a mother gives when her children are misbehaving in public. Now that look means 'please help!'"[5]

It Might Be Difficult to Keep Track of a Discussion

Some people with Alzheimer's have difficulty communicating due to problems tracking discussions. It is important to have one's hearing evaluated, since diminished hearing makes it harder to effectively track conversations. Hearing loss can often be remedied with hearing aids, but a person with memory loss has to remember to wear them!

More often with Alzheimer's, difficulty tracking conversations is due to memory loss and challenges remembering what someone has said. Conversations often move at a quick pace and it may take your mind longer now to process information and to form a reply. You may want to respond to something that is said during a conversation, but by the time you are ready to contribute your comment, the topic has changed or moved on. One man with Alzheimer's expresses appreciation for the pace of conversation in his support group: "Here we can go slow enough to honor each other's words."

Memory loss can also contribute to challenges in recalling content that may be referred to during conversation. Friends and families must learn to make adjustments. One woman says:

"One of the major challenges for me was to help them speak differently to me. My husband said to me, 'Boy I can't wait until Thursday, can you?' and it's like, 'What's Thursday?' I don't have a clue. I've had to teach them to say, 'I'm looking forward to Thursday when we'll see the Joneses—won't that be nice?'"[6]

For some people, it can also become more challenging to understand language. This is known as *receptive aphasia* and can contribute to problems with conversation. You may hear perfectly well, but your brain may not always interpret the meaning of what you hear. In an attempt to help you understand, others may speak more loudly to you, even though your hearing is not the problem. A more effective strategy is for others to rephrase their message to you using different words. Shorter sentences that convey one thought at a time are also helpful.

It is harder to track conversations when there is competing noise or activity. Alzheimer's can limit the brain's ability to separate sounds, so it can be helpful to limit distractions when you are in a conversation. Stop anything else you may be doing, turn off the television or radio, slow the pace, and look directly at the person you are talking with.

Smaller Social Gatherings May Be Easier for You

Conversations in social situations with large groups can be difficult for many people with Alzheimer's. Most people have experienced feeling left out of a conversation. Maybe people were discussing a topic you knew little about, so you weren't comfortable chiming in. Perhaps others spoke up more quickly or assertively, so you quietly deferred to the more talkative ones in the group. Or you were trying to form your thought clearly before you spoke it, but someone interrupted and changed the subject before you had a chance to contribute.

While these experiences may not be the norm for most people in typical conversations, they become increasingly common in a person with

Alzheimer's. It can be helpful for friends and family to remember their own experiences with similar situations so they can develop greater sensitivity to any difficulties you might have in group discussions.

Despite possible challenges, you may enjoy the dynamics and energy of group conversations. Perhaps you do not have significant communication challenges or are accustomed to larger groups and feel at home with animated conversation. Regardless of how you participate, you may enjoy the group and being included in the activity. However, some people find that smaller, quieter groups in which one person talks at a time are more relaxing and rewarding.

"I'm Still Here!"

Some people with Alzheimer's discuss feeling like they are being ignored or talked about in their presence as if they weren't there. This is a common complaint in the doctor's office when the physician may talk with your care partner, but not directly to you. This can also happen in social settings, when others make erroneous assumptions about your communication abilities. Barb describes how people defer conversations to her husband:

> "Some people, when my husband and I are together, refer to me as 'her,' not us or them or you two. It's like I'm there but they can't see me…And it's so aggravating. I want to stick my tongue out and say, 'I have Alzheimer's but I can still comprehend and speak for myself most of the time.'"[7]

As more people become outspoken advocates about the experience of living with Alzheimer's, they are changing common stereotypes about the disability and making both their presence and voice known. There may still be instances, however, when you feel disregarded during conversations and it is important that you and your loved ones let others know that you still deserve to be acknowledged and spoken to directly.

Keep Talking!

People with early-stage Alzheimer's vary considerably in their experiences with communication challenges. You may not relate to many of the issues discussed in this chapter, or you may identify with all of them. However, it can be helpful for you, your family, and your friends to know what is common to the Alzheimer's experience so you can make adjustments as needed. Regardless of the kind or frequency of your symptoms, it is important to stay connected to others and engaged in conversation in whatever way is meaningful and enjoyable.

Questions for Discussion

- Do you have any challenges with communication? If so, what are they?
- Are there responses from others that help you to communicate more effectively? Are there responses that hinder your communication?
- Do you ever find yourself avoiding communicating with others? If so when?
- When are you most comfortable communicating with others?

Suggestions for Improving Communication

- If you are open with others about your diagnosis, they are more likely to understand the reason for any communication difficulties and feel more at ease.
- Friends and family need to understand that your pace in conversation might be different. When you speak up, you may be referring to something that was discussed a few minutes ago because it took you longer to process your thought and get it out.
- Body language is a form of communication. You may look more tense, sad, or withdrawn but not express yourself with words. Likewise, you may become more sensitive to the body language of others. You and your loved ones can try to be more aware of any body language during communication.

- Participants of CoffeeHouse, an early-memory-loss support group for people with Alzheimer's in Ann Arbor, Michigan, advise families to:

  - Slow your speech.
  - Keep it short and to the point, one idea at a time.
  - Face me when you talk. Eye contact helps to get my complete attention.
  - Pause once you say your thoughts. Let me take the time to think through what you said to me.
  - Let me finish what I am trying to say. It takes a little longer, and sometimes it takes a lot longer!
  - Take the time to help me get my thoughts out. Ask me questions to help clarify my thoughts. Ask me if you can help find the words.
  - Please be patient. If you're tense, remember that I feel your tension, too.[8]

Chapter Nine

Helpful Tips for Managing Memory Loss

Memory loss is the primary symptom of Alzheimer's disease and is sometimes referred to as *amnesia*. You may have difficulty recalling the time, date, or appointments; where you put things; how to carry out routine tasks; or how to stay organized. You could forget someone's name or the plot of a movie or television show. The unpredictable nature of memory loss, especially in the early stages, can be confusing for you and your loved ones. "There is no rhyme nor reason to my problem," Sheila writes. "I can't even say, 'Well I remember these kinds of things, but I have a hard time remembering those kinds of things.' There's no neat pattern. Today I may be fine and then tomorrow, not so fine."[1]

> *"I try to maintain a sense of humor. Laughter helps me be more forgiving of myself."*

Although there is presently no way to reverse Alzheimer's-related memory loss, many individuals and their families develop creative ways to manage the effects of early-stage memory loss on daily life. As you read this chapter, you may find that you are already using some of the suggestions provided, or you may have your own to add.

General Principles of Managing Memory Loss

As you learn ways to manage your memory loss, you and your loved ones can consider the following general principles and strategies:

- **Break tasks into small steps.** It is easier to remember how to do something when it is done one step at a time. Finish one step before starting the next. For example, if you are trying to clean your desk, take one drawer or stack of paper at a time and finish sorting it before moving on to the next section. If you're doing yard work, finish raking before you start watering. Trying to do too many steps of a project at once can increase confusion.
- **Pay attention when you are trying to remember something.** Excess stimulus can interfere with attention and memory. For example, if you are trying to read while the television is on, or if you are having a conversation with someone while you are trying to pay a bill, your mind is trying to focus on too many things at once. Alzheimer's makes multi-tasking difficult. If you give close and undivided attention to something, you might remember it better.
- **Practice repetition.** When you are trying to learn a new activity or maintain the ability to perform a well-learned one, practice the activity over and over in the same way until it becomes familiar. Repetition may improve your ability to learn and recall. Be easy on yourself, though. Practice does not always make perfect. However, establishing familiar routines can be a helpful part of managing your memory.
- **Use multiple brain functions to help with remembering.** Memory is processed in multiple areas of the brain. The more regions of your brain that you use, the greater your potential for remembering. For example, when you watch a program on television, talk about it with someone afterward. This stimulates multiple areas of thinking and can

help with memory. "I make a point of watching the nightly news," says Barbara. "It's not always fun, but my husband and I talk about the issues that they discuss, and I think it's good for my brain."

- **Get adequate sleep.** Sleep is required to "consolidate" memories, a process that moves short-term memories into long-term storage. It is important to make sure you get adequate sleep each night and that you rest during the day if needed to restore your mind and body. Bert tells his friends in his support group, "I take a nap every afternoon. I kick off my shoes at about 2 o'clock and get some rest. I wake up refreshed and my mind feels clearer."

- **Your attitude can influence how well you cope with memory loss.** Alzheimer's symptoms can be extremely frustrating. If you become irritated trying to complete a task or remember something, try to take a break from the activity or your thoughts. Many people with Alzheimer's say that stress or anxiety worsens their memory problem. Phil advises: "If I can't remember something, I just stop, relax, give my mind a rest, and eventually it comes back to me. If you can't remember something, try to take a few deep breaths, let it go, and chances are, it might come back. But then again, sometimes it doesn't!"

- **Adjust your expectations of yourself.** Give yourself more time to do things, eliminate distractions, take one step at a time, and ask for help if needed. And most important, don't be too hard on yourself! You have a medical condition that impacts your thinking and functioning, and you are doing the best you can with a very challenging situation. Despite your best efforts to remember a piece of information, learn something new, or accomplish a particular task, you may not always succeed. You will be able to cope more effectively if you can be patient with yourself. Mark says, "I try to maintain a sense of humor. Laughter helps me be more forgiving of myself."

In recent years, many people with early-stage Alzheimer's have shared their specific strategies for coping with memory loss in support groups, at educational workshops or conferences, in essays they have shared with the public, in meetings with their healthcare providers, and in daily interactions with friends and family. The following tips and words of advice are paraphrased from this accumulated wisdom.

Strategies for Staying Organized

Memory loss can interfere with the ability to keep track of times, dates, appointments, and other important information. Many people cope with these challenges by developing systems for staying better organized and oriented:

- I write lists and notes to myself, but I just use one or two large yellow notepads that are easy to see and easy to find. I keep these pads in the same place. Small pieces of paper end up all over the place and I forget to look at them!
- I keep important information in my wallet like my address, phone number, and my medication list. My wife made a duplicate wallet for me because I lose it sometimes, and this way I have a spare until the other one is found.
- We keep a large desk calendar with appointments and activities listed on it. Right next to it is a clock that tells the time, day of the week, and date. I look at the clock for the date and then check the calendar for the day's plan. I cross off the days as they pass.
- I can't figure out a calendar very well these days, so we use a dry-erase board in the kitchen. Each day my daughter writes down the day, date, and any reminder notes or appointments for that day. I can only handle one day at a time.
- I keep a comprehensive day planner with me (I call it my brain) that has all of my schedules, appointments, and a calendar. It's attached to my purse so I have everything in one place. I always used one at work, so it's a familiar system for me.
- I keep a large pad of paper attached by a string to the phone. I write everything down when someone calls so I have the information for my daughter when she gets home.

- I have a watch that also has the date on it. I can press a button on the watch and it says the time out loud.
- I pick up the newspaper each day to read the date.

There are many other daily activities that may be disrupted by memory loss and require creative problem solving:

- I do the laundry on the same day each week. I wash everything in cold water so if I don't get the colors and whites all sorted out right, I don't end up with blue underwear.
- Every morning I feed my dog at the same time as I eat my breakfast. If I don't do it then, I may forget to feed her or feed her twice. She won't tell me if I've already fed her. She'll just eat again!
- When I'm cooking, I check off each step in a recipe to keep track of the steps I have completed. I put out all of the ingredients that I will use for the recipe and then as I use each ingredient, I put it away.

Strategies for Remembering Where You Put Things

Most people with Alzheimer's misplace things, and sometimes often. One woman says, "One of the problems with having such a bad memory is the unbelievable waste of time spent looking for things or having to retrace my steps altogether."[2]

- I keep a special basket in the living room where I always put important objects that I tend to lose, like my keys, glasses, or wallet. That way I'm less apt to forget where I put them.
- I have a pegboard in the garage where all of my tools hang. I outlined the shape of each tool on the board with a black marker, so when I take it down, I know exactly where to put it back. If I don't put a tool right back after I use it, I'll never find it again!
- Get rid of excess stuff! If you have less clutter, you have less to lose, and it's easier to find things.

- If I can't find something, I just let it go for a while. Sometimes I find it when I stop looking for it, or sometimes I just get over it because I forget what I was looking for!
- Sometimes I pray, "Dear God, just help me find it!"
- My daughter finds everything. I ask her where something is, and it works!
- I confess that I often blame someone else when I can't find something. I think I know where I put it, but I'm convinced somebody else moved it! That somebody was usually me, so my suggestion is to not go around blaming other people.
- I always forget where things are. It's just a lifestyle now, and beating myself up about it doesn't help. It's a nuisance for my family and me, but you have to keep your sense of humor because it's no one's fault.

Strategies for Remembering Names and People

Some people acknowledge that they have always had a poor memory for names or faces, but with Alzheimer's, it is not unusual to forget the names of people you know well.

- I keep a photo album with pictures and names of significant friends and family. I try to look at it often to refresh my memory.
- If I engage a person in conversation long enough, something they say may jog my memory about their name or who they are.
- My family and I have a strategy. If we are in a conversation with someone, they cover for me by repeating the person's name while we're all talking together. Sometimes they'll give a few casual introductory remarks to prompt my memory about the person.
- If my husband and I run into someone I know and should be able to introduce him to, he quickly introduces himself first and then the person introduces herself back and I'm saved the embarrassment of not remembering her name!
- I hope there is another person in the group who knows the person's name and uses it. I just listen and wait.

- I introduce myself, even if we might already know each other, and hope that the other person does the same. Sometimes I just say, "Hey buddy, how are you doing?"
- I just tell people that I have Alzheimer's and that I'm bad at remembering names. It's about as good an excuse as you can get for forgetting someone's name!
- I just call everybody "honey!"

Concern about forgetting names and faces can be greater at group events, reunions, or family gatherings where there are multiple names and faces to remember.

- If we're going to a family gathering, sometimes before we go, we'll look at pictures and go over names so I can rehearse which name goes with which person.
- I was at a reunion and I just looked at everyone's nametags. Thank goodness for nametags!
- My wife and I recently went to a wedding and we asked to see the guest list before attending. This gave me time to go over the names of the people I should know. My wife and I repeated the names and talked about these people in the weeks before the event and it made the event less stressful.
- I make sure to get a lot of rest before a group event and I limit my alcohol consumption during the event. I don't think as well when I'm tired or fuzzy from alcohol.
- If there is music at a group event or party, I take a break from the pressures of conversation, get out on the dance floor, and have a good time!

Forgetting names or faces is common in early-stage Alzheimer's. If you have not told family members or friends about your Alzheimer's, you may feel more stressed trying to pretend everything is fine when it isn't. If you let others know about your memory problem, you may feel less embarrassed if you forget a name or a face. People are often understanding of memory lapses that are due to a medical problem. Bobby is candid with her friends, saying:

> "I tell them, 'I keep forgetting what your name is. And I keep forgetting what street I live on.' They'll laugh at me, which is good. Maybe not for them, but it is for me. I'm funny sometimes!"[3]

Strategies to Prevent Getting Disoriented or Lost

One of the more frightening experiences of Alzheimer's is becoming disoriented or lost in familiar places. Memory loss or changes in vision and perception can make the familiar look unfamiliar. Many people with early-stage Alzheimer's continue to value their independence, and a few helpful strategies can increase your autonomy and safety. There are three nation-wide programs for people with memory loss to help get you home safely if you become lost, disoriented, or injured and can't find your way. These programs involve wearing an identification bracelet, necklace, or global positioning device that is linked to a national database that police or paramedics can access if you need assistance: Medic Alert/Safe Return (888-572-8566 or www.medicalert.org/safereturn), Project Lifesaver (877-580-5433 or www.projectlifesaver.org), and Comfort Zone (877-259-4850 or www.alz.org/comfortzone).

Other suggestions from people with Alzheimer's include:

- My son and I take a walk together every morning. We take the same route for the same amount of time. If I go alone, the route is familiar and I'm more likely to find my way back home. If I'm gone longer than usual, he knows to come looking for me.
- I like to take walks by myself, and I drive places alone. So far, I'm OK, but sometimes my husband comes with me. He doesn't give any directions. He just wants to make sure I still know where I'm going. I don't really like it, but I know he's right to be concerned.

- I carry an ID card with me when I go out because it tells me who I am and where I live.
- I got to know the neighbors on my route so I can ask them for directions or help if I become lost or disoriented.
- My wife bought me a voice-activated cell phone that she reminds me to carry. It's easy to use because I don't have to remember numbers to call someone. If I'm on a walk or out doing errands and I don't come back on time, she can call me. We taped my home phone number to the back of the cell phone so someone can call my wife if I need help.
- I don't go out of the house by myself in extreme weather. When I'm too warm or too cold, I don't think as clearly, and I don't want to get lost somewhere in bad weather.
- When I walk into a department store, I pay close attention to landmarks. I'll note whether I walked in past the jewelry counter or the men's department. It helps me find my way back out.
- I carry a miniature tape recorder to record reminders to myself. I'll record where my car is parked, or directions to get somewhere. It's so small that it fits easily in my pocket.

Not all of these strategies may be useful to you, or perhaps a strategy works one day but not the next. It is possible, however, to develop helpful strategies for dealing with memory loss. Brainstorm with others and you may come up with your own unique strategies to add to the list.

Questions for Discussion

- When does your memory loss give you the most trouble?
- Which of these memory-loss management strategies do you use?
- Which strategies do you want to try?
- Do you have other strategies to add to the lists?

Suggestions for Developing Your Own Memory Management Strategies

- Make a list of the main ways that memory loss interferes with your daily life. Under each problem, list some possible strategies you can use to try to manage it more effectively.
- Involve loved ones or friends in your memory management strategies. Teamwork is often more effective than trying to go at this alone.
- Talk with other families who are dealing with early-stage Alzheimer's and brainstorm about different strategies together. Much can be learned by sharing your experiences with others.

Chapter Ten

Dealing Effectively with Other Symptoms

Alzheimer's can affect different regions of the brain that are responsible for thinking, behavior, and functioning. Although memory loss is the primary symptom of Alzheimer's, changes in problem-solving abilities, mood, vision, and motor coordination can create different challenges in daily life. This chapter provides a brief overview of some methods for managing other symptoms commonly described by people with early-stage Alzheimer's.

> *Each person experiences Alzheimer's differently. Some symptoms could be minimal, while others might be more persistent.*

Managing Disrupted Sleep

There are many ways that Alzheimer's can disrupt sleep patterns. Some people report having vivid and disruptive dreams with the start of a prescribed Alzheimer's medication. It is important to discuss any sleep disruption with your doctor to see if the timing, dosage, or type of your medication needs to be adjusted. Do not take any over-the-counter sleep medications without consulting your doctor, as compounds in these common sleep aids can increase confusion and other problems with thinking in people with Alzheimer's.

Sleeping too much or too little can be a symptom of depression. Other sleep disorders, such as sleep apnea (interrupted breathing during sleep that includes loud snoring or sudden gasping) or restless leg syndrome, can interrupt sleep patterns. Discuss any change in mood or sleeping patterns with your doctor so you can be evaluated and treated for any sleep disorders.

Sleep is also influenced by our circadian rhythm. Circadian rhythm is an internal biological clock that helps to regulate your sleep and wake cycle. This rhythm can become disturbed, resulting in irritability, confusion, too much sleeping during the day, or getting up at night thinking it is daytime. Circadian rhythms are sometimes stabilized by adequate exposure to light. Try to get exposure to bright sunlight or bright indoor light throughout the day as it may help you to sleep better at night. When possible, go to bed at the same time each night to develop a routine and keep your bedroom dark, quiet, and at a comfortable temperature. When one man was getting up too early each day, he and his wife bought a large, easy-to-read digital clock for his bedside table to alert him to stay in bed until at least 6 am.

Avoid excessive napping during the day as well as drinking caffeinated coffee, tea, or soda after noon, as these behaviors can disrupt sleep. Try not to watch disturbing news or other media before bedtime, and instead enjoy soothing music or a video with calming imagery or content.

If Routine Tasks Become Difficult

You might have difficulty carrying out the steps required to complete a familiar task. For example, you may get out the sewing machine to hem some pants, but then you can't figure out how to proceed. Or you may go to mow the lawn, but find that the lawnmower is now more confusing to operate. This problem is called *apraxia* and it can result in frustrating experiences.

Apraxia can interfere with basic daily activities. For example, some people have difficulty with the steps involved in getting dressed. Dressing requires a great deal of memory and other thinking processes. You must be aware of the season and the general temperature of the day in order to pick appropriate clothing. You have to recall and judge whether you have already worn something multiple times and whether it is clean or not. You have to remember where articles of clothing are kept and in what order they need to go on. You must also have the physical coordination to manage small buttons, zippers, snaps, or hooks. Alzheimer's can interfere with the brain's ability to transmit messages necessary to coordinate our actions. For example, David tells friends in his support group about challenges coordinating his hands as he's trying to button his shirt: "I know what to do, but my hands just won't do what I want them to!"

When you add up the steps and thinking processes involved in getting dressed, this routine activity becomes a complex task. Some suggestions for making dressing easier include:

- Simplify! Put your spring and summer season clothes away during fall and winter months to reduce confusing choices. Get rid of old clothes that you rarely wear to limit clutter in closets and drawers. Assemble outfits in closets or drawers so you reduce the number of choices you have to make about matching shirts with slacks or skirts with blouses.
- Lay out your clothes the night before so they are ready the next morning.
- Consider wearing more pull-on pants or pullover shirts if buttons or zippers are a problem. Keep all but the top buttons on button-up shirts closed so you can simply pull the shirt over your head.
- Give yourself extra time. Having to rush is likely to increase stress and confusion. Cary Henderson writes:

> "When someone wants me to hurry up, I can't hurry up—there's no way to hurry up. The hurrier I get, the behinder I get, and I think that's pretty much for anybody with Alzheimer's. We can't be rushed because we get so doggone confused we don't know what we're rushing about."[1]

Adapting to Difficulties with Reading and Writing

It is common for people with Alzheimer's to have difficulty reading, since memory loss can affect concentration. Some people report that by the time they have read to the bottom of a page, they have forgotten the content that was at the top. The following suggestions may be helpful:

- Read shorter articles in newspapers or magazines. If you can finish the article or story in one sitting, you may be more able to keep track of the content. One man says, "It takes longer for me to read than it used to, but I guess I have the time, so it's OK. Reading is always a discovery because I learn something new or get lost (I definitely get lost!) in the story. But I tend to read short stories or magazines now, so I can usually keep track pretty well."
- Read a paragraph over until it becomes familiar. Sometimes repetition can help memory.
- Discuss what you have read with someone else. Discussing the material may prompt your memory and help you retain the information longer.
- Read about topics or articles that interest you, such as hobbies you enjoy, your previous professional work, places you have traveled, or specific current events. When you are interested in something, you pay better attention and might more effectively store and retain memory.
- Although it takes effort, try making a few written notes about some of the facts, names, or content in what you are reading. Writing notes may help to prompt your memory, and you can refer back to them as needed.

Some people experience perceptual and visual changes in the brain that make it difficult to interpret written letters or words, or to track lines of text. Large-print books are often easier to read. Audiobooks are a popular solution that eliminates the task of reading by allowing you to listen to recorded books or magazines from a CD or cassette tape. Contact your local library for more information about this valuable program or contact the National Library for the Blind and Physically Handicapped (202-707-5100).

It is also common for handwriting to change over the course of Alzheimer's. Writing is a complex task involving multiple regions of the brain. Some people report that their writing is smaller or harder to read. One woman describes her creative solution to the problem: "I have a lot I want to say in a letter, so my friend has offered to re-write my letters for me or she writes while I dictate." Another woman shares that she has a drawer full of cards with printed messages on them. She picks the right card for the right occasion and signs her name. Simplifying your written messages to others can lessen your frustration. A lot can be said with just a few words!

Some people have hand tremors or find it hard to coordinate a pen. Those who are familiar with typewriters or computers may continue to type, although sometimes more slowly. One man says, "I was an engineer and had exquisite handwriting, but now I find I have terrible penmanship, so I use a computer and a large font size. Thank God for spell check! I fought it for awhile, but it's something you've got to accept."

Understanding "Sundowning"

The term sundowning is used to describe the restless, confused, or anxious feelings some people with Alzheimer's experience during the late afternoon or early evening. The hours around dusk can be particularly disorienting or unsettling and can create problems for you and your care partner.

If you think about your previously familiar routines, the time around sundown may have been a time of transition. Many people were accustomed to leaving work and heading home or may have been busy preparing a meal for a family coming in from a day at work or school. Memories of these patterns can be deeply ingrained and lead to a feeling of increased restlessness or anticipation at sundown.

Living with Alzheimer's symptoms can also be tiring, and you may feel more fatigued toward the end of the day. Fatigue can increase irritability and confusion and may contribute to sundowning. Alzheimer's can also affect your ability to interpret what you see. Changes in light toward the end of the day can produce shadows or dim conditions. Shadowy shapes may look like people, or dimly lit rooms may look unfamiliar in the fading light. This can be frightening or disorienting and lead to confusion.

Not everyone experiences sundowning, and those who do may find it to be an unpredictable symptom. Some days may be just fine, while others bring on anxious feelings. If you experience problems with sundowning, consider the following suggestions:

- Try to keep your home well lit as evening approaches. This can help with the transition from daytime to nighttime.
- Do not take on challenging activities in the later part of the afternoon or evening. A quiet visit with a friend, soft music, or helping to prepare the evening meal may help to pass this transition time more smoothly.
- When weather allows, some people find that an evening walk or slow drive around the neighborhood eases restless feelings. It is important to have someone with you during these late afternoon outings for both companionship and safety.
- If you have routinely disruptive problems with sundowning, contact your doctor. Sometimes medicine can be helpful for managing persistent anxiety of distress.

It can be difficult to read about possible symptoms, or it could be reassuring to know that if you have them, there may be creative solutions for managing them. It can be helpful to talk to others who share these same experiences. It is common to hear people with Alzheimer's discuss the importance of being patient with yourself and maintaining a good sense of humor. These may be the most valuable suggestions of all.

Questions for Discussion

- Do you experience any of the problems described in this chapter? If so, which ones? Have you discussed them with your care partner or doctor?
- What strategies have you used for coping with any symptoms?

- Have others suggested any ideas for managing symptoms? If so, how have you responded to these ideas? Has your response helped you or your care partner to cope more effectively?

Suggestions for Managing Other Symptoms

- Each person experiences Alzheimer's differently. Some symptoms may be minimal, while others might be more persistent. Although you may try to conceal problems or hope they will just go away, tell your care partner or doctor about them so you can find effective ways of managing these challenges.
- Brainstorm with your care partner or others about creative ways to cope with symptoms, and make a list of your own strategies.
- Contact your local Alzheimer's organizations for educational materials. Many resources are written for your loved ones so they can learn effective ways of working with problems when they arise.

Chapter Eleven

Improving the Safety of Your Home Environment

Symptoms of Alzheimer's can impact your safety at home, but there are effective ways to minimize hazards. This chapter reviews some common areas in which early-stage Alzheimer's symptoms can pose safety concerns and offers simple suggestions that address them. Your doctor may be able to prescribe a home safety evaluation through a home health agency so a nurse can visit your home and provide recommendations to reduce your risk of in-home injury. This can be an effective way to begin thinking about home safety and taking precautions as needed.

> *Certain home safety precautions can maximize your independence and reduce your risk for injury.*

Preventing Falls and Staying on Your Feet

Many studies suggest that people with Alzheimer's are at increased risk for cuts and bruises, sprains, and fractured or broken bones as a result of a fall. Falls can happen in the home or out in the community. They can be

---

caused by tripping, slipping on wet or uneven surfaces, losing your balance, moving too quickly when distracted or upset by something, or misjudging the height of a curb or step. Alzheimer's can affect your ability to judge both depth and distance. Something may look closer or farther away, or taller or shorter in height than it really is. Other eye conditions, such as macular degeneration, cataracts, or outdated glasses or contact lenses can complicate visual problems, so it is always wise to have your eyes examined if you or your care partner notice any problems with vision or spatial relationships.

Some people with Alzheimer's become restless and feel the need to move about or stay on the go. This restlessness can affect movement and concentration, and it can increase risk for falls or accidents. Others may also have symptoms associated with Parkinson's disease. These can include a shuffling walk and some inflexibility, also called *rigidity*.

There are many ways to take precautions that can reduce your risk of a fall:

- Use night-lights in the bathroom, bedroom, and hallways. One man says, "Sometimes I feel like I can get lost in my own house, so night-lights help to point the way."
- Make sure any stairs inside or outside your home are well lit. Consider putting brightly colored tape or paint on the edge of each stair to better define each step. Install and use a handrail, if needed.
- Install grab rails in the shower and by the toilet. Use rubber bath mats or textured adhesive strips in the shower or tub to reduce the risk of slipping on wet surfaces. Consider sitting on a shower stool or bench while bathing if you have a problem with balance.
- To avoid tripping, keep furniture and other significant objects in the same place. Keep telephone and electrical cords and excess clutter out of pathways. Remove loose throw rugs.
- Wear sturdy, low-heeled shoes that fit snugly.
- Store frequently used objects within reach so that you can avoid using step stools or chairs to reach things.
- Consider using a cane or walking stick for balance and for judging

distances or heights of curbs and stairs. Slow down when approaching curbs and stairs.

- Avoid walking alone on busy streets. Memory loss combined with too much noise and stimulus can affect both concentration and judgment and increase risk for accidents.
- Exercise regularly to maintain muscle flexibility and strength.

Make sure you let someone know if you have fallen! Some injuries are not outwardly or immediately apparent. You may not be aware that you have injured yourself, and you could need medical evaluation.

The Complications of Cooking

If you have memory loss, remembering the multiple steps involved in cooking a meal can be challenging. Leaving out an ingredient of a recipe may not be the end of the world, but forgetting you have left the stove on and burning a pot or pan could result in a dangerous fire. Alzheimer's can decrease your sense of smell, making it harder to detect when something is burning. Many people who live with a spouse or family member are grateful when someone else begins to help with the cooking. But, if you live alone or want to continue cooking, consider the following tips:

- Set a timer for anything you are cooking and limit your use of the stove. One woman says, "I only use the stove now to boil water for coffee. I make myself stay at the stove until the water is boiled, and then I turn it off right away so that I won't forget."
- Use the microwave whenever possible. Although items can still be overcooked or burned, there is less risk for fire. One woman says, "I just use the microwave now instead of the stove. When I burnt the second teakettle, my daughter said that was enough!"[1]
- Label all of your kitchen cupboards and drawers to indicate their contents so you are less apt to misplace items or put them away in unusual places.

- Make sure you have a smoke alarm installed in your kitchen.
- If your care partner does most of the cooking, try to stay involved by washing the produce, stirring the soup, or tossing the salad. These activities can increase your interest in food and also help to maintain important skills.

Overcoming Cabinet Clutter

A general principle for coping with Alzheimer is to establish methods of organization. If you have fewer things to sift through, you greatly improve your chances of remembering and finding whatever you are looking for. Sometimes Alzheimer's makes it harder to distinguish one item from another or to clearly identify objects. There are ways to improve organization and to ensure your greater safety:

- Do not store prescription medicines in the same cabinet as vitamins, supplements, or over-the-counter medications (such as aspirin). Prescription medications should be stored separately so they are not confused with other pill bottles.
- Check expiration dates on prescriptions and throw out expired ones.
- Separate routine medications from those you take "as needed" to minimize the risk of taking excess medications.
- Use a weekly pillbox for your routine medications to track whether you have taken them.
- If you have toiletries that look somewhat similar (tubes of toothpaste and denture cream or shampoo bottles and liquid soap dispensers) label the containers with an indelible-ink pen to avoid confusion.
- Secure all cleaning products and other potentially toxic substances in their own cabinets, separate from any other contents. Label the cabinet "hazardous."
- If you have dietary restrictions, you may be less able to remember them. Label foods in your cupboards that you should not be eating or separate those foods so they are not easy to reach.

Dismantling or Removing Weapons

Weapons pose a significant safety hazard for people with Alzheimer's. Even in the early stages, symptoms can interfere with the memory, judgment, and motor skills (coordination) needed to effectively maintain or safely use a weapon. Some people are very defensive about any discussion of their weapons and are attached to them for security or recreational reasons, or because a collection may have historic, personal, or family significance. If you have any weapons in the home, the following precautions are important for maintaining the safety of yourself and others.

- Lock any weapons securely in a cabinet or other storage container.
- Remove any ammunition or keep blanks in any weapon.
- Make weapons inoperable by removing the firing pins.
- Pass weapons on to the family members who may appreciate them.

Avoiding Getting Locked In or Locked Out

The following general safety precautions can help ensure that you are able to enter and exit spaces safely as needed:

- Eliminate locks on bathroom doors. If you fall in the bathroom and have locked yourself in, it is much harder for someone to help you if needed.
- Consider leaving a set of your house keys with a trusted neighbor. It is not uncommon to forget or misplace keys, and this could result in getting locked out of the house.
- Plan how you will exit your house in the event of a fire or emergency. Avoid interior locks or deadbolts that require a key to open the door. It may be difficult to remember where the key is or to use it effectively under stress.

Taking Caution in Hot and Cold Weather

In many parts of the country, winter months pose significant challenges for staying warm and healthy. *Hypothermia* occurs when a person's body temperature drops dangerously low from exposure to cold. Low body temperature can contribute to serious health conditions, including heart attack, kidney problems, or liver damage. People with memory loss must take extra precautions to avoid circumstances that could lead to hypothermia, including becoming lost or disoriented while outdoors alone in cold weather. Also, some people may forget to dress warmly enough or forget to turn up the home thermostat to a comfortable temperature and become dangerously cold without realizing it.

Warm weather can be a welcome relief, but it may pose its own challenges. Dehydration can increase confusion or disorientation, as can heat stroke. Due to memory problems, you may simply forget to drink enough fluids. Some people with Alzheimer's lose sensitivity to thirst and are unaware when their body is signaling the need for liquids.

- In warm weather, fill a quart-size water bottle with water or fruit juice every morning and drink from it throughout the day. If you have forgotten whether you've had enough fluids at the end of the day, check the bottle. If it's empty, that's a good sign. If it's still full, drink up!
- An acute onset of confusion or change in your functioning should be medically evaluated to make sure you are not dehydrated.
- Avoid going outside alone in the hottest part of the day or during severe weather.

Since each person experiences Alzheimer's differently, it is important to adapt your environment to address your specific concerns. However, general home safety precautions can help you to maximize your independence and reduce risk for injury to yourself or others.

Questions for Discussion

- Have you or your care partner observed any ways that Alzheimer's has affected your safety in the home? If so, what modifications have you made to improve safety?
- Would you be reluctant to take any of the safety precautions suggested in this chapter? Is so, why?
- What ideas do you have for maximizing your independence and safety in your home?

Suggestions to Consider When Evaluating Home Safety Needs

- Consult with your doctor or other healthcare provider about any specific symptoms you may have that could interfere with home safety.
- Ask your doctor to request a home safety evaluation through a local home health agency. Many insurance policies will pay for this visit.
- Think about your daily routines and evaluate ways to reduce any safety risks. Read, download, or order this helpful free booklet: *Home Safety for People with Alzheimer's* at 800-438-4380 or www.nia.nih.gov/Alzheimers/Publications/ homesafety.
- Make sure that you and your care partner have an effective disaster and evacuation plan, in case of a fire or natural disaster. Read, download, or order this helpful free booklet: *The Calm Before the Storm: Family Conversations about Disaster Planning, Caregiving, Alzheimer's Disease, and Dementia* at www.thehartford.com/calmbeforethestorm.

Chapter Twelve

Making Decisions about Driving

This chapter addresses one of the more heated issues for people living with early-stage Alzheimer's. Many individuals and their loved ones struggle to understand the effects of memory loss and other symptoms on driving performance and at what point it may no longer be safe to drive. Some individuals are not very troubled by the decision to stop driving, while others describe the driving controversy as one of the most difficult issues they face. Given how significant the loss of driving privileges can feel, it is important to understand the potential impact of Alzheimer's on driving skills.

"There seemed to be a point of confusion on my part as to whether I was that bad or could just watch it until something happens."

This chapter addresses some of the most frequently asked questions about driving when you have Alzheimer's and provides suggestions for managing decisions about this challenging issue.

How Can Alzheimer's Affect My Driving?

Memory loss, disorientation, and changes in vision and perception can cause drivers with Alzheimer's to misjudge distances, forget the rules of the road, or have delayed reaction times when making the multiple quick decisions needed to drive safely on freeways or around town. Alzheimer's may also affect concentration and coordination. Memory loss can make you feel more frustrated or anxious in stressful situations. You may drive too slowly and create a safety hazard because it takes more effort to focus on your driving or to remember the directions to your destination.

It is common for people with Alzheimer's to get lost even while driving in familiar places. Jean recalls a frightening episode:

> "Recently I was driving in a familiar area, but I had gone farther than I usually go. There were buildings on either side, but nothing seemed to be open. So I went back and forth and back and forth and I was afraid to move more because then I really wouldn't know where I was. It was like a nightmare. I finally saw a door on somebody's building that was halfway open so I asked for directions. Then I was OK when I knew what to do next. But the fear is that I'm lost forever. I think it's a fear of being stranded."[1]

Do People with Alzheimer's Get In More Accidents?

Research indicates that drivers with Alzheimer's are more likely to get into motor vehicle accidents. These accidents vary from mild fender benders to tragic events involving loss of life when the driver with Alzheimer's makes a very serious and unexpected error in judgment. Some people voluntarily give up driving after encouragement from their doctor, family, or friends, or after a frightening spell of disorientation or an accident. Others refuse to let go of the steering wheel, and their driving can become a significant life-threatening personal and public safety hazard.

Will I Lose My Driver's License Because of My Diagnosis?

Laws concerning Alzheimer's and driving vary considerably from state to state. It is uncommon to have your license automatically revoked due to a diagnosis of Alzheimer's or a related disorder, but you may need to be evaluated to make sure that you can continue to drive safely. In some states, physicians are mandated by law to report your diagnosis to the Health Department or the Department of Motor Vehicles if they think your symptoms could affect your driving abilities. You are then asked to take a written and a driving test to evaluate your ability to drive safely. In other states, your physician may conduct his or her own evaluation and, based on the findings, make a recommendation about your driving. Some physicians order a driving performance evaluation through an occupational therapist or a center that specializes in testing drivers with specific medical conditions. Sometimes a concerned family or friend may make a report or request that you be evaluated, but many families look to the physician to assume this responsibility in order to avoid being the target of their loved one's potential anger or resistance.

Some people with early-stage Alzheimer's continue to be safe drivers for a limited time while others, due to the kinds of symptoms they are experiencing, are at risk of making dangerous mistakes and should stop driving. The symptoms of Alzheimer's can vary from person to person, so consult with your doctor about the potential impact of your symptoms on driving performance. Your physician should also be familiar with the laws or procedures in your area for drivers safety evaluations.

How Can I Know if I Am an Unsafe Driver?

You may not be the best judge of your own driving. Sometimes a friend or family member notices problems before you do. A retired air force pilot with Alzheimer's writes:

"There seemed to be a point of confusion on my part as to whether I was 'that bad' or could just 'watch it' until something happens. After all, I'd been driving for all of my adult life and only had a few minor accidents. How could I be expected to give up my keys without a fight?"[2]

Many people with Alzheimer's have clean driving records and resent that others are telling them to stop driving, especially when there may be worse drivers on the road. However, it is smarter to quit driving while you can still take pride in your driving record than wait until you have an accident that results in a serious injury, a lawsuit, or death. Vaughn Collins laments the loss of driving, but respects his wife's judgment about his safety. He writes:

"The loss of freedom to drive is one of the harder facts of Alzheimer's life. I feel that my hands-on driving skills are as good as ever, but not my memory of how to get from here to there. I have made the decision that Rosella's feelings are the final word. If she is not relaxed with my driving, she becomes the driver, and that is almost always now."[3]

Look for the following problems when you are driving, or listen if someone points them out to you:

- Forgetting how to get to familiar places or becoming disoriented while driving can indicate serious changes in memory or concentration.
- Misjudging distances, such as driving too closely to others, not staying within your lane, or having difficulty parking, can be due to vision and perception changes.
- Failure to follow traffic signals, such as running stop signs or red lights, stopping at a green light, or forgetting the meaning of other traffic-related signs.
- Poor decision-making, including not using turn signals, forgetting to look in your mirrors, weaving across lanes, becoming confused at

four-way intersections, or not yielding to traffic when necessary.

- Driving significantly more slowly than the speed limit, which can be hazardous.
- Losing your temper or becoming easily frustrated can signal that you are getting overwhelmed by the multiple demands and stressors of driving.

If I Get in an Accident, Can I Be Sued Because of My Diagnosis?

If you have a valid driver's license, you have the legal right to drive. However, if your symptoms are affecting your driving abilities and you do not voluntarily stop driving or seek retesting for driving safety, you may be at fault or at risk of getting sued if you are in an accident. Someone could charge that you knowingly drove or that your family let you drive with a disability that put you and others at risk for injury. Check with your car insurance company to make sure that they would cover you in an accident or keep you insured if you were driving with a disability that is known to affect driving safety.

Some people try to appeal the revocation of their driving privileges and want a second chance at passing driving tests or evaluations. This is usually not advisable. While symptoms of Alzheimer's can be stable for quite some time, they generally do not get better. If your driver's license has been revoked due to the effect of symptoms on driving safety, this situation is not likely to improve with more time or repeated efforts. It is wise to accept the decision and stop driving before you injure yourself or others. If you continue to drive, you and your family need to show good faith in keeping up to date on the effects of Alzheimer's on your driving performance. It is strongly recommended, for legal and ethical reasons, to be voluntarily retested or medically reevaluated every six months for safe driving.

If I Have to Stop Driving, How Will I Cope?

You may have a wide range of feelings if you give up driving. Feelings might pass quickly as you adjust to this loss, or they could last for some time and be difficult to resolve. Some people feel depressed or demoralized when they can no longer drive and many experience a loss of freedom, spontaneity, and control. You may have to conform more to your driver's schedule or go places that you don't want to go when en route to your own destination. The increased need to rely on others can feel frustrating or inconvenient. Bobbi says, "Maybe I'm wrong to even try to do anything other than have people take care of me. But somehow that doesn't suit me, and I think that's why I miss driving."[4]

While it is important to acknowledge these feelings, you must focus on your remaining choices and abilities. If you are not doing the driving, you can still have some say in the destination. You may not always be able to go exactly where or when you want to, but if you can schedule some activities and outings in advance, this gives others more time to plan transportation arrangements. Friends and family are often willing to provide transportation. Some urban areas have door-to-door transportation services specifically designed for people with disabilities. Other sources of transportation can include volunteer church groups, social service agencies, or senior centers.

If you have to ride along for someone else's errands or stops along the way, take along a magazine to read, listen to music or an audiobook, take a nap, look at the scenery, and try to avoid becoming a backseat driver when others are doing their best to get you where you want to go. Carol lives alone and writes:

> "Yesterday I was driven for the first time by my designated driver, a 70-year-old retired neighbor who is thrilled to have a few extra dollars now and then. I can tell you that it was not difficult at all. In fact, it was a relief not to have the worry of whether my response time is what it should be, getting lost, or becoming confused. I highly recommend not putting off getting out from behind the driver's seat. We must understand that it isn't just our life, but the lives of others we could be jeopardizing."[5]

Some people feel angry or betrayed that others doubt their ability to drive. Sometimes it is difficult not to take the whole issue of driving personally. However, Alzheimer's is only one of many medical conditions that affect drivers safety. You are not being singled out, and many people of varying ages and disabilities also need to stop driving. If you are reluctant to burden a friend or family member with your transportation needs, consider that others would probably rather assist with your transportation than see you drive unsafely or withdraw from your activities.

Some people voluntarily give up driving and take pride in making a responsible sacrifice for the safety and well-being of others. Others begin to feel that driving is too stressful and are relieved to let someone else take over this responsibility. After much consideration, the air force pilot quoted earlier concluded:

> "There is really no use for me to argue about the issue of driving. When I consider the liability issues for myself, as well as my caregiver, it simply isn't worth the risk to continue driving. I must consider the safety of passengers, pedestrians, and other drivers as well as innocent children and myself…There are some good things to contemplate, though. There is only one insurance bill, I have maintenance and upkeep on only one car, and I now have my own chauffeur and companion. Also, I now see things as a passenger that I was never able to see as a driver."[6]

Questions for Discussion

If you are driving:

- Are you driving with the current approval of your physician or Department of Motor Vehicles? If not, what steps can you take to be evaluated for safe driving?
- Has anyone suggested that you have any of the problems with driving discussed in this chapter? If so, how have you responded?

- At what point would you think it is no longer safe to continue driving?
- If you have to give up driving at some point, do you have other means of transportation in place when needed?

If you are no longer driving:

- Was the decision to stop driving your own or someone else's?
- Have you accepted why you can no longer drive? If not, what would help with that acceptance?
- How have you managed your transportation needs? Have these solutions been effective?
- Have there been any positive outcomes from no longer driving?

Suggestions for Dealing with Transportation Issues

- Read, download, or order this helpful free resource: *At the Crossroads: Family Conversations about Alzheimer's Disease, Dementia, and Driving* at www.thehartford.com/alzheimers.
- Explore transportation options in your community through Alzheimer's organizations, senior services organizations, or volunteer groups.
- If you have an extra vehicle that is no longer being used, sell it and put the proceeds into a special personal transportation fund to hire drivers as needed.
- Consider walking shorter distances when possible. Walking is excellent exercise and can be a pleasurable way to get somewhere. One man tells his peers, "I advise you and anyone else who has a problem with driving to remember that you have two legs. Maybe you need new shoes, but go ahead and get them!"[7]

Chapter Thirteen

If You Live Alone

It is difficult to estimate the number of people around the world who are living alone with Alzheimer's. Although many people manage on their own for quite some time with limited support, personal independence must be balanced with responsible attention to safety, emotional and physical well-being, and the needs or concerns of your loved ones.

If you live alone, you may have some concerns about your own well-being. Or, you may think that you are managing fine and resent that others are questioning your self-reliance. It is common for people to have varying degrees of tolerance for risk. What poses a safety concern for one person may not be a problem to someone else. However, changes in your memory and thinking could affect your ability to judge how well you are doing on your own, and conflicting opinions could create tension between you and concerned others.

> *Arranging for help as needed can support your independence and allow you to live on your own for a longer period of time.*

Many factors are involved in decisions about living alone, including the sort of assistance that may be available to you, your finances, your family and community supports, and your safety. This process of evaluating your living situation may be gradual, or a more immediate decision may be needed to help you maintain your well-being or avoid risk to yourself or others. This chapter gives an overview of issues to consider when living alone, and provides ideas for how to get help as needed to maximize your safety and independence. If possible, sit down with a trusted family member, friend, or professional and go through the questions posed in this chapter. If you have differing opinions about whether you should live alone, try to consider feedback from others who care about you and may be concerned.

Food Preparation

Are you able to make a list of what you need at the store and manage your grocery shopping? Can you prepare well-balanced meals? Have you burned pots or cooking items on your stove? Is there spoiled food in your refrigerator that could be harmful to eat? Do you drink enough fluids? (Dehydration can worsen symptoms of memory loss and confusion.) Are you maintaining adequate weight?

There are a number of ways to manage food preparation and nutrition. Try to buy small amounts of food at a time to avoid spoilage, and focus on non-perishable foods if possible. If you no longer drive, there may be a grocery store in your community that could deliver food to your home. You can work with a family member or friend to place an order. Most communities also have home-delivered meal programs, such as Meals on Wheels. These services can provide up to two meals a day and considerably reduce meal-preparation responsibilities. If you continue to cook, it is often safer to use a microwave rather than the stove. "I no longer use the stove without being supervised so that's the biggest problem for me staying alone," says Audrey. "I actually had two fires. I don't mean burning things, I mean actual fires."[1]

There are many nutritious frozen meals that can be prepared in a microwave. Use a microwave to boil water or get an electric teakettle that automatically turns off when the water has boiled.

Managing Medications

Are you able to keep track of when to take your medications? Are you forgetting to take them or taking them too frequently? Are there expired medications in your home or medications that have not been refilled as needed?

Medication management can be very challenging for people who live alone, and an effective system is critical. Most people rely on a weekly medication container that separates their medicines into time slots for each day of the week. More elaborate medication dispensers have timers or voice notifications that alert you to take medications. Other people with memory loss have systems of separating morning, afternoon, and evening medications on different shelves of their medicine cabinet or checking off medications on lists after they take them. It may be easier to remember to take medications if they are next to your refrigerator or on the table where you eat.

Sometimes family members or other assistants make routine medication reminder phone calls or drop by daily or weekly to make sure medications are being taken. While some medications have limited side effects if you miss a dose or accidentally take them twice, others can have very serious health consequences if not taken consistently and specifically as directed. If you live alone and have health issues that require strict medication adherence, it is not wise to manage your own medications. A few lapses in your memory could result in a serious risk to your health and your independence.

Managing Finances and Paying Bills

Are you able to maintain your checkbook, write checks, and pay bills? Have you discovered any overdue bills or accidentally thrown any away? Has your power, water, or phone ever been turned off because you didn't pay the bill? Can you calculate the correct change in purchasing transactions at stores? Have you given any money to fraudulent or exploitive phone or mail solicitors?

It is common for people with early-stage Alzheimer's to have difficulty with numbers. People frequently find it is more challenging to write checks and manage the checkbook or to keep track of their bills and payments. You may want to continue managing your finances but benefit from some assistance so that serious errors can be avoided. One woman who lives alone was relieved when she hired a bookkeeper. "With the checkbook, I knew when it was time to give it up," she says. "Let somebody else do it. This charming woman is just great with my checkbook!"[2]

Some people opt to keep all of their incoming bills and important mail in one place on a desk or table and then work with a family member or professional bookkeeper once or twice a month to help with organization and payment. Others find that a successful solution is to have all utility and other routine bills submitted directly to the bank and paid from your checking account. This ensures that your bills are paid accurately and on time and eliminates any worry about keeping track of them. If you receive monthly income, this can usually be directly deposited into your bank account and eliminates the risk of you misplacing a letter or check. (See Chapter 26 for important information on legal and financial planning that can help to ensure that your finances are managed if you are unable to continue doing this on your own.)

People with early-stage Alzheimer's who live alone are at risk of being financially exploited by phone and door-to-door solicitors. The following steps can reduce risk:

- Get your phone number registered on the National Do Not Call List by calling 888-382-1222.
- Post a "No Solicitation" sign on your front door.

Attending to Personal Hygiene and Grooming

Are you bathing or showering safely and adequately? (Bathrooms are a common place for falls or other accidents.) Are you experiencing any medical conditions such as skin rashes or urinary tract infections that could indicate difficulty maintaining good hygiene? Are you doing your laundry as needed?

We often take for granted the ease of dressing and grooming, but these tasks are actually quite complex. Memory loss, diminished sense of smell, and trouble with problem solving can all contribute to challenges with the multiple steps involved in grooming and hygiene. Some people with early-stage Alzheimer's have few problems in these areas, while others who live alone may unintentionally begin to avoid these tasks by bathing less or wearing the same outfits repeatedly. Grooming and hygiene are sensitive and personal issues, and if others notice changes in your habits, they may be reluctant to discuss their concerns with you. If a family member or close friend does bring up the subject, try to appreciate that they are concerned about your dignity and welfare. It may be helpful to have someone assist you with weekly laundry and with sorting your clothes for the upcoming week. Home safety modifications in the bathroom can reduce risk of injury during bathing, which is especially important when you are living alone (see Chapter 11).

What Would You Do in an Emergency?

If there is an emergency in your home, such as a fire or you have a medical problem, do you know what number to call and how to use the telephone? Do you have any problems with balance or vision disturbance that could increase your risk of falling? If you smoke, do you remember to extinguish cigarettes? Are there any burn marks or holes in your furniture upholstery, carpets, bed linens, or clothing? Do you remember to lock your doors at night before going to bed?

People who live alone need to be able to problem-solve during an emergency. Have emergency numbers posted next to each phone or, when possible, also program them directly into your phones. Make sure that you have working smoke alarms installed throughout your home and that all exits to your home are free of clutter in case you need to get out in a hurry. Try to work with your neighbors to establish an emergency plan in case you need assistance or have to evacuate from your home.

Some people find that a personal emergency response system is an excellent form of security when living alone. These systems include a bracelet the size of a large watch or a necklace that your wear 24 hours a day. The bracelet or necklace has a button on it that you press in case of an emergency. This activates the emergency response team and they call you at home to determine your need. If you are unable to get to the phone, paramedics are immediately sent to your house to investigate. Some programs also include routine phone safety checks. Call your local hospital, senior center, or Alzheimer's organization to find out what personal emergency response programs are available in your community.

The Responsibilities of Home Maintenance

Are you able to manage the routine upkeep of your home? Is it relatively free of excess clutter that can accumulate and create safety problems? Can you manage any equipment needed to clean the house or do yard work, such as a vacuum cleaner or lawn mower? Are you able to coordinate home repairs by calling a plumber or electrician?

For some, taking care of their home is a matter of personal pride, and maintenance responsibilities are meaningful and rewarding activities. For others, the tasks can become overwhelming. It can be difficult to remember all of the steps required in home maintenance, and repairs that require more complex problem-solving can become challenging. Hiring a housekeeper for thorough and routine housecleaning or having a family member assist can be an effective way to manage home upkeep. This affords you the chance to do lighter daily housekeeping while being assured that comprehensive cleaning and maintenance will be taken care of. If you live alone, it is important to have a list of well-recommended people you can employ or rely on to help with home repairs as needed.

The Risk of Social Isolation or Withdrawal

You may have been living on your own for quite some time and be accustomed to it. Or, perhaps you are recently widowed, separated from a family member or friend, or alone due to a recent move to a new location. People who live alone need to pay extra attention to maintaining social contact with others. With the onset of memory loss or other symptoms of Alzheimer's, it can become harder to organize social activity. Friends may need to take more initiative and help keep you connected to others.

If you live in a neighborhood where others are well acquainted with you, there may be a comforting sense of community and security in the daily interactions with your neighbors. For many people, however, it is hard to rely on neighbors as the primary source of companionship or assistance. Some communities have social service agencies that exist specifically to help seniors or persons with disabilities who are living alone, and these agencies can be valuable resources in helping you to build or maintain connections with others and get assistance as needed. For more information, you can contact Eldercare Locator at 800-677-1116 or www.eldercare.gov.

The Benefits of Care Managers

Care managers are social workers, nurses, psychologists, or other professionals who work with seniors or persons with disabilities to help them live successfully in their homes. There is usually a fee for these services. Many care managers have expertise in addressing the needs of people with early-stage Alzheimer's who are trying to maintain their independence. Care managers help to determine what services you need and then coordinate those services in the home. They can screen and hire home help as needed and oversee the quality and effectiveness of any assistance or services. If living at home is no longer the best option, care managers can make recommendations for other living arrangements and help with any move or transition.

Care managers can work with individuals, couples, or whole families and be an invaluable member of a care team. They can also provide relief to families who live some distance from their loved one with Alzheimer's and are thus unable to coordinate needed resources and services. Referrals for professional care managers can be found through local senior centers, Alzheimer's organizations, or community social service agencies. You can also contact National Association of Professional Geriatric Care Managers at 520-881-8008 or www.caremanager.org.

When to Consider Other Living Arrangements

There will come a point when it is no longer advisable to live alone. This may be due to the safety issues and other considerations discussed in this chapter, or you may have other needs or circumstances that necessitate a change of living arrangements. Perhaps you are lonely or would like more company. One woman says, "I think living alone at this point now is something that is just plain old. I want some interaction with people."[3]

People with Alzheimer's who live alone eventually either bring people into their home to help them, or they move in with a family member or a care community that provides assistance. You and your loved ones must decide which option works best for you, and everyone may not be in agreement. Sometimes discussing the situation with an objective outside party, such as a doctor, social worker, or care manager, can help to sort out the options. Some people worry about bringing strangers into their home, and it is important to do thorough screening of any person you may consider for this position. You may find reliable and trustworthy companions through word of mouth at churches, senior centers, through neighbors, or a referral from a friend or care manager.

Some people are unable to find consistent or compatible help in the home. Others may benefit from the stimulation, security, and convenience of a long-term care community. It can be very helpful to investigate potential assisted living or residential care communities and determine what might be an affordable or reasonable alternative if needed. If moving in with a family member or friend is an option, discuss any concerns about this plan now so that any move in the future happens more smoothly. Try to make your preferences known about alternate living arrangements so you have can have some control in this significant decision.

The questions to consider presented throughout this chapter may seem overwhelming, but if you or your loved ones have observed problems in any of the areas discussed, it is important to accept some assistance in the home or consider a different living arrangement. Accepting assistance does not mean giving up control of your life. On the contrary, arranging for help as needed can support your independence and allow you to live on your own for a longer period of time. (See Chapter 16 for a more detailed discussion of accepting help from others.)

Questions for Discussion

- Are you and your loved ones in agreement about your living alone? If you do not have close friends or family nearby, has anyone else expressed concern about you? What are their concerns?
- What steps can you take to ensure that you can continue to live alone safely and independently if that is your preference?
- If you are unable to live alone at some point, what would be your next step? Would you prefer to get more help in your home or move to a different living arrangement?

Suggestions to Consider When Living Alone

- Decide who is on your support team, including family, friends, professionals, and hired assistants who can help you maintain your well-being at home.
- Acknowledge any concerns about your living alone. Don't wait too long to get needed help. If you have an emergency, or accident, or begin to jeopardize your own safety, you risk having to leave your home prematurely or against your will.
- Take one step at a time and start early so you can hire help gradually and increase the assistance as needed. This allows you to build trust with others and get accustomed to new people in your life.
- Go with a friend or family member to look at options for retirement or care communities, so you know what is available in your community.
- If you plan to move in with family in the future, make any house renovations or modifications now so that the house is ready when needed.

Chapter Fourteen

Understanding and Managing Your Feelings

The experience of Alzheimer's or a related disorder can lead to a wide range of feelings that vary from person to person. Some feelings may be familiar and consistent with your previous temperament, while others may surface as a result of challenges related to memory loss and other symptoms. Many feelings that you experience in your daily life will continue to be satisfying and enjoyable, and you can maximize these feelings through effective coping. This chapter gives an overview of some of the more challenging feelings that can accompany Alzheimer's and offers suggestions for managing them if they arise.

> *Your approach to challenges makes a big difference in how you get through the tough times.*

You Could Feel Depressed or Discouraged

Many people with Alzheimer's experience symptoms of depression, including sadness, hopelessness, lack of initiative, sleep disturbance, and changes in eating habits. Given the many challenges associated with Alzheimer's, it is understandable to feel discouraged sometimes. "I get aggravated with myself and I can cry a lot easier than I can laugh," says Bea. "I've lost my feeling of self satisfaction that I was capable of doing things, and I resent it a little bit. But I'll live through it."[1] Feelings of diminished self-worth or self-esteem can be discouraging. One woman in the video, *Alzheimer's Disease: Inside Looking Out* states, "I still would like to be treated like a person, you know, because I'm still a person whether I do it wrong or right."[2]

Everyone has down spells when it is hard to cope, but your approach to challenges makes a big difference in how you get through the tough times. Thaddeus Raushi makes a point of focusing on his strengths instead of his symptoms:

> "I continue to take advantage of my capabilities to build on what I can do and not simply bemoan what I can't do. Certainly I miss the abilities that I am losing; daily I am reminded of the losses. Some days I am down and disappointed and not full of life. Yet, when I am down, I allow myself to feel this way; I don't try to pretend the feelings aren't there. To do so would not be true or healthy. But I have a choice to stay in that place or move on. In moving on I accentuate those abilities and qualities that I do have and also work at using them to compensate for ones I do not have."[3]

Suggestions for managing depressed or discouraged feelings include:

- Examine any discouraging thoughts that may be contributing to your depression, and try to replace them with more hopeful ones. Take a day at a time and try to find the bright spots in each day. Focus on your abilities and make use of them.
- Participating in a support group can help ease feelings of discouragement and provide an important sense of belonging and community. "When I came to the group, I was very depressed, but it's going away,"

says one group member. "Being with other people with the same problems helps…being able to talk about it and work on it."[4]

- In many parts of the world, winter brings shorter days and limited sunshine, which can increase risk for depression. If you feel more depressed in winter, consider using special light bulbs or light boxes in your home that can compensate for the lack of natural sunlight and help to elevate mood.
- Your doctor may prescribe an antidepressant medication if symptoms of depression are acute or persistent.

It is Not Uncommon to Feel Angry or Irritable

The experience of memory loss and other symptoms can be very frustrating, and there will likely be times when you feel angry or irritable. Although some people with Alzheimer's are less bothered by symptoms and maintain an even or easygoing temperament, many have feelings of anger or frustration that can vary in intensity and duration. One man says:

> "Sometimes I feel so exasperated! I just want to explode. My wife is grateful that my rage doesn't get vocal and fall out all over her. She marvels at this all the time. She is perpetually thunderstruck that I can retain any humor in this at all. I'm a little thunderstruck that she can find a little humor sometimes, too. But, screaming and hollering and pulling my hair out is not going to help."[5]

Situations that can provoke anger or irritability include when:

- You feel rushed or pressured to do something.
- You have difficulty doing something that you previously did with ease.
- Someone jumps in to help you with something that you want to do yourself.
- You feel a loss of control.

- There is too much activity, noise, or stimulus going on at once.
- You can't find the right words to express yourself, or you lose your train of thought.
- You feel tired, vulnerable, or frightened.
- Your dignity or pride is threatened by someone else's comments, actions, or your own confrontation with Alzheimer's symptoms. One woman says, "I get so frustrated at this disease. I have had lots of successes in my life until this disease hit…Now I do well at nothing. I get so frustrated, it comes out as steam at the people around me."[6]

You may also be more sensitive to expressions of frustration or irritability in others, and sometimes this can set off your own anger. Robert Simpson writes:

> "I have more difficulty dealing with anger in a constructive way than I once did. If somebody gets angry, or I feel they are angry, I feel it emotionally. Before, I could have worked it through my head and not taken it personally or reacted too much. I could have understood. Now I have an emotional response that is less clear, and it takes me longer to set it in perspective…I get more upset than I would have at one time."[7]

People with Alzheimer's who are more irritable are also more likely to be depressed. A medical problem resulting in pain, infection, or discomfort can also increase irritability until the problem has been effectively treated. It is important to discuss any increase in anger or irritability with your doctor.

Suggestions for managing anger and irritability include:

- Try to recognize triggers for anger and frustration so that you and your loved ones can limit situations that provoke conflict. For example, members of a support groups in the Okanagan region of British Columbia, Canada, offer this insight and advice to families: "I may say something that is real to me but may not be factual. I am not lying, even

if the information is not correct. Don't argue; it won't solve anything."[8]
- Daily physical exercise can release tension.
- Get adequate rest. Disrupted sleep and fatigue contribute to irritability.
- The company of a pet can ease tension. One man says, "My little dog takes the edge off. He doesn't talk back, but he communicates with me. He senses when I'm upset, and he comes over and puts his head in my lap."
- Frequent feelings or expressions of significant anger may be lessened by medications aimed at reducing irritability. Talk with your doctor if you or your loved ones think you may benefit from medicine.

You May Feel Frightened or Anxious

Symptoms of Alzheimer's can be frightening at times and result in anxious feelings. You may not be able to count on all of your abilities like you used to, and it could require time to adjust personal expectations of yourself. You may also rely more on others for reassurance when you are in challenging situations. "Because information overload and crowds confuse me, I often feel fearful," one woman says. "This makes me want to cling to my husband. I need him to be a buffer zone between a confusing world and me."[9] For some, being separated for any length of time from the people they count on can be stressful. Alzheimer's can distort your sense of time so that your care partner's hour-long absence feels like forever.

Others feel anxious because they think too much about the future and its challenging possibilities. Perhaps you benefit from learning as much as you can, but for most people, this is not emotionally helpful or constructive. Elizabeth wisely states, "Don't overreact. Get support. Try to avoid getting sick with worry."[10] No one can predict the future, so people living with Alzheimer's often advise a "one day at a time" approach to ease anxiety. When you only focus on your fears, you lose sight of all of the positive and hopeful things available to you in your life now.

You may feel frightened because you are unsure of yourself and are cautious about your abilities. It can take courage to acknowledge fears, and it is wise to respect your feelings and share them with others so that they can be more understanding. Jean says:

> "Even if I don't want to do something because I'm scared, that's just as important. A lot of people won't allow themselves to be overwhelmed by something. But for me, I think 'Don't do this—it will only make it worse.' I'm scared for a good reason. Maybe not somebody else's good reason, but my own."[11]

Suggestions for dealing with anxious feelings include:

- Try to work with your care partner to identify the situations that provoke your fears or anxiety. If you routinely pretend that everything is fine when it isn't, others will not know how to partner with you to reduce these upsetting feelings.
- Robert Davis, a retired minister, writes about his own fears and provides wise advice to family members: "There is a way to help…but it is definitely not by reasoning…This is the time for comfort, reassurance, a soft touch, and a gentle voice with soothing words…As soon as my wife is aware that I am in one of these states, she embraces me…She asks me to tell her about what was bothering me. As I talk about it, the panic subsides and I am made aware that I am in touch with reality again…"[12]
- Focus on your breathing during anxious times. Breathe slowly and deeply to calm yourself down.
- Some people can distract themselves from anxious feelings by listening to calming music, exercising, participating in an enjoyable activity, or talking with others. Find what works for you so you have coping tools to use as needed.

You Could Feel Suspicious or Tend to Blame Others

Most people can recall times in their life when they have felt suspicious or have unfairly blamed others for their problem. Perhaps you couldn't find something and were convinced someone took it until you realized it was right where you last left it. Maybe you suddenly noticed less money in your bank account and suspected theft until you remembered the extra expenses you had incurred that month. Perhaps you were at fault in a car accident but wanted to blame the other driver. Although anyone can feel suspicious or defensive sometimes, the experience can be more frequent for people with Alzheimer's.

Memory loss can contribute to feelings of suspicion. If you can't remember whether you did or did not do something, where you put a missing object, or whether you discussed an issue with someone, it is easy to assume someone else is at fault or is not being truthful. You may also feel more unsure of yourself and less trusting of others as a result of Alzheimer's symptoms. One man in Great Britain says:

> "I was the most happy-go-lucky fellow. I used to go down to the club and pub and drink whisky. Now I don't want to go out. And I don't want anyone coming in here. I weigh people up. I'm watching them. In my position, the way that I feel, I don't have trust. And I was never like that."[13]

Feelings of fear, vulnerability, being left, or being left out are often at the root of suspiciousness. Robert Davis describes his suspicions about money:

> "I saw what was happening in me and I could name it at the time as paranoia. However, even though I saw it happening to me, I could do nothing to stop the feelings. I worried particularly about money. There was no reason to worry about money…I had such a great fear. I doubted any financial security. It was irrational, but I could do nothing to control the fear. After several months of constant reassurance from my friends and my wife, I am better able to deal with these paranoid feelings."[14]

Sometimes there is a seed of truth in your feelings that grows out of proportion and gets generalized to other things. For example, you may have loaned money to someone who never paid you back. Now you fear others are stealing from you. Maybe your spouse had to go on a business trip or visit a family member for a few days, but you forgot about the plan and now you think loved ones are going to leave you for good. Maybe you had a housekeeper who stole something from you years ago, so now you won't let anyone come into your home to help. Alzheimer's can make it difficult to distinguish the past from the present, and this can result in confusing feelings of uncertainty.

Consider the following when trying to manage feelings of suspiciousness:

- If you get stuck on a suspicious thought or fear, try to get your mind off of it with a pleasant activity, conversation, or other way to focus your attention.
- Your feelings of suspiciousness can be difficult for your loved ones because you might unduly blame them for problems. They will need their own support from professionals or other care partners on how to provide reassurance, not take your accusations personally, and learn strategies for dealing with your specific fears.
- If you feel someone is trying to physically or emotionally harm you or take advantage of you, talk with your doctor, social worker, or other healthcare provider about the problem so you can receive assistance or protection as needed.

My "Get Up and Go" Is Gone!

You might have a harder time getting motivated to do things. This is often referred to as reduced initiative, or increased apathy. For example, you or your care partner may wonder why you don't go out and water the yard, pick up that book of crossword puzzles, call a friend, or do something else on your own. Reduced "get up and go" is often the result of changes in the brain that affect *executive functioning*—that is, the ability to focus, make decisions, problem-solve, or multi-task. You may have difficulty with the steps necessary to begin or accomplish a task, or you could be challenged or fatigued by the focus and decision-making required to participate in an activity. These are common complaints that can affect your motivation. Having Alzheimer's means it takes more energy and concentration to do things that you previously accomplished with ease.

Some people have reduced motivation because they fear they can no longer do routine activities successfully, or their care partner has automatically assumed all responsibility. If others have eliminated certain responsibilities or activities from your life, you may feel less initiative or drive. Linda Raymer writes:

> "There is a fine line between realizing I must give up a certain part of my life in order to make my life easier and giving up everything entirely…Each small occurrence by itself is not significant. It occurs so gradually, but eventually, nothing remains. Therefore there is no motivation…The caregiver is well-meaning in trying to protect their loved one from any harm to themselves physically and emotionally…Perhaps there would be motivation if there was an alternative to the losses."[15]

If you are not able to replace lost activities with meaningful ones to take their place, you may have a reduced sense of purpose.

The following suggestions may be helpful:

- Adjust your expectations of your daily activity level as needed and set reasonable goals. Focus on fewer activities but allow for more time.
- Partner with someone to accomplish a task or an activity rather than giving it up entirely.
- Develop a routine, make a schedule, and try to include a few specific activities each day, such as a walk, lunch date, or housekeeping responsibility.
- Do one thing at a time and one step at a time.
- Keep hobby or activity materials in plain sight as visual reminders.

Put puzzle books on the coffee table; hang the dog's leash by the front door; designate a special workbench or table for easy access to a project.

Developing Positive Attitudes and Coping Strategies

In the publication *Don't Make the Journey Alone*, a group of Scottish individuals with Alzheimer's or a related disorder write, "The best person to help you cope with your new life is yourself. It is your attitude that is going to be really important."[16]

Positive attitudes and coping strategies are acquired and used throughout life. Some coping strategies may be familiar methods that you have used at other challenging times, while others may be new skills that you are developing to deal with memory loss and other symptoms. It is never too late to develop helpful coping strategies. The following suggestions are offered by people with Alzheimer's and speak to the diverse ways people manage their feelings.

- **Get your mind off Alzheimer's.** Staying busy can be a helpful way of coping with feelings. One woman says, "I don't think about Alzheimer's! I have lots of other wonderful things to think about—children, grandchildren, reading, walking, eating, and chocolate!" Another man agrees with this approach and says, "When my mind is on something else, I can't think of myself, so I stay busy." Some people feel that they have plenty of meaningful activity, while others struggle to find ways to fill the time (see Chapter 17).
- **Learn to let go.** There may be times when you struggle to do something or make something go your way to no avail. Try to stop the battle and take a break. Joe laughs when he says, "Look, half of having smarts is knowing what you're dumb at. Don't beat your head against the wall."
- **Don't give up on life.** "I am not giving up," says Francine. "There are other things besides having Alzheimer's."

- **Think positive.** Brian McNaughton writes, "If we passively shut up shop in the early stages of our disease and just concentrate on what a horrible card fate has dealt us, then we deserve to be miserable and should be ashamed of making the lives of those who love us so stressful. Instead, look for those opportunities to stray from the beaten path. Leave your dark rooms and open your hearts if you have trouble opening your minds. It's hard at first, I must admit, but it gets easier the more you try."[17]

- **Focus on your remaining strengths.** One man says, "Look, Alzheimer's is only part of what I am, not all of who I am." You have many remaining abilities and positive qualities. Acknowledge them and make the most of them.

- **Give and receive support.** People with Alzheimer's support one another by participating in groups, social programs, email chat rooms, or other activities. The opportunity to share with others who understand can ease many challenging feelings. Glen says, "You can always talk with your friends. We help each other out. We'd all be the first to help each other."

- **Learn to accept that you have Alzheimer's.** Retired physician Dr. Donald Rhodes reflects on his own process of coming to terms with his diagnosis:

> "There's the intellectual acceptance part, and the emotional acceptance part, and you fuse them together, for wanting to survive. People want to survive. They want to continue. With this, if you want to survive and continue, you have to accept. Then try and make realistic plans and accommodations for your life."[18]

Learning acceptance does not mean that everything always goes smoothly, but this approach can help you move forward and live your best. Bea says:

"I have accepted the Alzheimer's, but I have to gripe some! I don't spend a lot of unpleasant hours or days thinking about it. I go on with my life and do what there is to do. And my life is pretty darn good, all things considered."[19]

Questions for Discussion

- Which feelings in this chapter do you identify with? How are you managing them?
- What coping strategies do you identify with?
- What other actions, strategies, or attitudes help you to cope?
- Do you have any attitudes or behaviors that interfere with your ability to cope?

Suggestions for Managing Feelings

- Try to acknowledge your feelings and share them with others, including your loved ones, friends, doctor, or counselor. Consider writing in a journal to release and process feelings.
- Write a list of your positive coping strategies and refer to it during difficult times. Also list any negative attitudes that interfere with your coping so you can limit them.
- Consider the coping strategies already noted by your peers. Focus on one at a time to determine if the strategy is helpful.
- Understand that Alzheimer's can have a mind of its own. You may not always be in full control of your feelings. Seek professional help if feelings become unmanageable or begin to interfere with quality of life.

Chapter Fifteen

The Benefits of Support Groups for You and Your Family

With the advent of earlier diagnosis, more people with early-stage Alzheimer's are meeting others through support groups. Early-stage support groups bring people together to share their thoughts, feelings, experiences, and knowledge with one another. The distinction of an early-stage support group is that participants are dealing with issues and concerns common to those who are newly diagnosed or only mildly to moderately affected by symptoms and interested in discussing their feelings and experiences.

> *"We learn from each other. Everyone has so much wisdom. We also get a lot of laughs in this group."*

"What Happens in a Support Group?"

The format and structure of early-stage support groups vary. Many groups are offered on a time-limited basis. The group may run for six to

---

twelve weeks and then end. Participants can then choose to continue meeting informally or, in some cases, follow-up groups are offered on a monthly basis. In other formats, groups meet weekly and are ongoing. Participants join the group and attend meetings for an unlimited period of time until the discussion topics are no longer meaningful to their circumstances or their symptoms advance and interfere with participation. Many support group formats also include separate meetings for an accompanying family member or friend so they can discuss issues relevant to care partners and share experiences or helpful resources.

Common discussion themes in early-stage support groups include: methods of coping with memory loss and other symptoms; the effects of Alzheimer's on social and family relationships; maintaining physical and emotional health; finding meaningful activity; participation in research and clinical trials; and driving and safety issues. Meetings might incorporate guest speakers, or participants may bring articles or other resources to share.

Although rare, some support groups are established specifically for people with young-onset Alzheimer's (under age 65) so they can meet with age-related peers. Younger people have concerns regarding early retirement, legal and financial planning, family issues, and social needs that may be different from people diagnosed in their later years (see Chapter 6). However, many support group members feel that regardless of age, they all have shared issues and can empathize meaningfully with one another about living with Alzheimer's.

"I'm Not Alone"

The diagnosis of Alzheimer's or a related disorder can leave a person feeling alone and discouraged. Upon coming to a support group, new members often comment that they never knew there were others facing the same problems. Most find a common bond in their willingness to acknowledge that memory loss and other symptoms are affecting their lives. Tom says:

"When you start out, you think you're the only one affected, and then in these groups, you find out there are others in the same situation. You come to a point where you aren't afraid of it, although you'd like to not have it. We're all unique here with Alzheimer's. It affects each person a little differently."

Another participant says, "It's my salvation to be able to go to a place and be around others in the same predicament. We can get out of the predicament for a while by being with a group of friends."

Knowing that you are not alone and that there are others living capably with symptoms can help ease feelings of isolation or worries about the stigma that can accompany an Alzheimer's diagnosis. One woman states, "You see that everyone is still the same person. We have difficulty doing things, but we're not lesser people."

"Problems Aren't as Drastic as They Used to Be"

Some people can come to terms with their diagnosis and gain perspective more effectively by sharing their experience of symptoms with others. Many support group participants are comforted when they share an experience with memory loss or another problem and find others in the group smiling and giving knowing nods in return. One group member says:

"The big thing for me was the fear of not knowing what was going to happen, the fright of mental confusion, the fright of what you hear about it [Alzheimer's], the frightening effect it has on your spouse and children. But learning more about Alzheimer's has helped. Groups like this are survival…I'm having less trouble with crying and being depressed. Problems aren't as drastic as they used to be."[1]

It can be helpful to see that life can go on, and the friendships that are formed in support groups often help to smooth the road ahead.

The sharing of mutual experiences can be equally helpful for care partners who are confused or frustrated by a loved one's symptoms. One participant of an early-stage Alzheimer's support group talks about his wife's participation in her concurrent care partner meeting. He says, "It's good for her to have a place to go to talk about me. And they all learn a lot from each other about how to best help us, so I'm glad she has a place to go for support."

The Importance of Feeling Understood

It can be hard for people who don't have Alzheimer's to fully understand the experiences of people who do. Many support group participants feel less self-conscious being with peers who share similar concerns. Peers are very understanding of memory loss and other symptoms, and support groups are a safe place to make a mistake. When asked what he most values about his support group, one man says, "The interaction—being here talking to everybody and being able to express myself without being criticized. We learn from each other. Everyone has so much wisdom. We also get lots of laughs in this group." Bernice comments, "The most important thing is to be able to be with people who have the same problems, and then if you want to say something, you can feel comfortable. We're all in the same boat." To which another group member responds, "Yes, and we're not sinking!"

The need for peer support and an outlet for feelings is worldwide and shared by a participant of a group in Grampion, North East Scotland, who says:

> "Having this illness is a lonely experience, even when you have a close family who gives you a lot of love. There is a part of me that they can't reach or understand, but when I'm with my buddies, I don't have that lonely feeling because they can understand me."[2]

The Value of Learning from Others

Many people attend support groups hoping to learn helpful information or coping strategies. Some participants bring newspaper or magazine articles to discuss with the group. With the growing influx of media information about Alzheimer's, it is helpful to have a place to go to obtain accurate information.

Most support group facilitators are professionals who can help to clarify information or find appropriate answers to questions as needed. Participants of an early-stage support group in Montreal, Quebec, reflect on their group experience:

> "It helped many of us discuss Alzheimer's more openly with family and friends, and we've learned about research, medication, and now we have a little more hope. Some of us have learned a few new tricks, too, like keeping a regular agenda, jotting down notes, and making other changes to help us remember things. It doesn't always work, but it helps to know there are some options."[3]

Care partners also experience the educational value of their support groups. Talking with other families about a shared condition helps to build community, and everyone can be more honest and at greater ease when discussing common experiences. Care partners also develop greater understanding of their loved one's symptoms and learn helpful tips for providing assistance as needed. Victor DiMeo, a retired psychologist with Alzheimer's joined a support group for himself and his wife. He says:

> "I'm a very caring person, and the support group brings me closer to other people. It makes me feel I want to do things for them and for myself. My wife also comes to the group at the same time and participates with the other spouses in their own group. I think she enjoys it. It's beautiful to see the changes in

people. By your action, somebody gets better. Because of your participation, somebody feels good again. Visiting the group makes me feel like I'm somebody. I'm alive."[4]

The Rewards of Giving to Others

Many people with Alzheimer's discuss the difficulty of not being able to do the things they used to do, including contributing to the lives of others in meaningful ways. Participation in a support group provides an opportunity to help others and can give meaning to the Alzheimer's experience. A support group member in Chicago says:

> "It is up to each member of this club to help the other who is failing. A pat on the back and a smile is all you need. At first I said, 'Oh well, what's the difference; my life is almost over,' but it isn't over. I think people who give their time to help others are fabulous."[5]

Some support group participants and their families form friendships outside of the group and enjoy socializing with one another through other activities or gatherings. These friendships can be a rich way to give and receive and can provide meaningful consistency through the ups and downs of Alzheimer's. Participants of a support group at the Long Island Alzheimer's Foundation in New York write:

> "A rich life is still possible, as we know from our laugh-filled yet serious meetings, as well as from the lunches with our new friends and spouses afterward. Who would think you could make new friends after you get Alzheimer's?"[6]

Overcoming Reluctance to Participate

It is not uncommon to have reservations about attending a support group. Often it is a concerned family member or friend who calls, looking for a group through which everyone can learn how to cope more effectively. Some people don't identify with the concept of a support group and question its value.

Frequently, however, a feeling of safety and belonging develops when participants discover they can share with one another and be understood. Les Dennis writes:

> "Support groups are probably good for most everyone, at least occasionally. I was never a fan of them, but when I went to my first group, I had just lost my right to drive, and I was pretty angry. I felt they were a bunch of strange people but I went along...we have developed a camaraderie that is deeply intertwined. We can talk openly. When one has a problem, all try to help. When there is a sickness, we console. The caring and concern is obvious and beneficial. We are also very funny. We laugh with each other, and we laugh at the disease. We often have a dark humor riding with us. All of us look forward to the weekly one-and-a-half-hour meeting."[7]

Bob overcame his reluctance to attend a San Diego support group and became a regular participant. He states with characteristic wry humor, "I like all of the people in my support group. I just wish I'd never met them!"

Support Groups Are Not for Everyone

Some people have never felt comfortable in group settings, have never been "joiners," or do not identify with the concept of "support." Others would simply rather not go to an activity each week that reminds them of having Alzheimer's, and do not think they could benefit from the experience. Perhaps you attended a support group, but did not have a positive experience. Maybe it was overwhelming, boring, or you felt you didn't fit in. You might have been uncomfortable seeing a participant who had more significant symptoms, or may not have felt the group was facilitated properly.

Support group attendance is a personal decision. Although caring others may encourage you to attend a trial meeting, no one should try to force the activity upon you. It is important that you have a choice. Your feelings about attending a support group may change in the future, so it is worth reconsidering the decision from time to time.

If You Don't Have a Support Group in Your Community

There are many regions of the world where people do not have access to early-stage Alzheimer's support groups, or participants have to travel considerable distance to get to one. This may be due to limited services in your area, or to community stigma surrounding Alzheimer's. Some regions of the country or some cultures across the world are not accustomed to the idea of "support" and may be more receptive to an early-stage group that is more education-based, where the focus is in receiving information and learning.

If you do not have a support group in your community and would like to meet others with early-stage Alzheimer's, contact your regional Alzheimer's-related organizations to see if they can help to start a support group. If they are not able, ask them to connect you with others in your geographic area who are living with early-stage symptoms. Sometimes families develop informal self-facilitated support groups or can involve a local senior center or religious organization as a sponsor. The Internet and email can also help families around the world to communicate with one another without having to leave home!

Questions for Discussion

- If you currently attend an early-stage support group, what do you gain from the experience? Is there anything that could make the experience even more meaningful? What topics are most interesting to you?
- If you do not attend a support group, why not? Are you comfortable

with your decision, or would anything help to change your mind?

- Have you ever participated in a support group for a different reason? If so, has that experience influenced your decision to participate in an early-stage Alzheimer's group?

Suggestions for Making the Most of Your Support Group Experience

- Attend more than one meeting to make sure you give the group a chance. Support group meetings can vary from session to session. Not every week will be equally meaningful, and the overall experience is what counts.
- Write down concerns, coping tips, or questions that arise for you during the week so you can take them to your support group meeting for discussion.
- If you have a concern about the content, facilitation, or another participant in your group, talk with your facilitator. Your feedback may help to improve the support group experience not only for yourself, but also for others. If you are not comfortable giving feedback, perhaps your care partner can talk with the facilitator.

Learning to Accept Help When You Need It

Alzheimer's symptoms can affect your ability to perform a variety of tasks or activities. What may seem like simple or automatic behaviors—doing the laundry, making a meal, driving, calculating change at the grocery store, or mowing the lawn—actually involves a complex series of steps that require considerable memory and problem-solving skills.

> *When you accept help, a task can be accomplished together and you are better able to exercise your abilities.*

Alzheimer's can disrupt your ability to do things that you may have previously taken for granted. There will be times when you need assistance, and learning to accept help when you need it is a constructive tool in maintaining your abilities and managing memory loss.

You May Have Mixed Feelings about Accepting Help

People have varied responses to the idea of accepting help. If you have a problem, it can be a relief to accept assistance. If you need support, it is reassuring to know you don't always have to persevere alone. Some find comfort in accepting help and feel strengthened by being able to partner with someone else to accomplish a task. Tom says, "I'm an expert at depending on my wife and daughters to keep me out of trouble, and that's a full-time job for them. I'm very lucky I have their love to keep me straight."

But the process of asking for and receiving help is not always easy. Perhaps you pride yourself in being independent and are uncomfortable when others get involved in your activities. Audrey, who lives alone, says:

> "One of the important things is being open about your circumstances and asking for help and, having said that, both of those things…are extremely difficult to do…You've got to trust and understand the people you're being open with and asking for help because I've seen too many cases where they overreact…so it's a scary process to open up."[1]

You may fear that others will jump in too quickly and take over your life. Yet, if you are not open to receiving some amount of help as needed, you may jeopardize your own safety or well being and lose even greater control.

Loved ones and concerned others also struggle to pace themselves and must learn to provide necessary help without being overbearing. Jeff sympathizes with his mother's reluctance to accept help. He says:

> "I've developed more empathy for what my mom must be going through. I'm a lot like her in some ways and I often ask myself, 'How would I feel if I were in her shoes. How would I react if that was happening to me?' and it makes me slow down sometimes. I can get going on my own track about what is right for her but I just try to pause a lot more now and that helps build the trust in our relationship."

"How Do I Know When I Need Assistance?"

Sometimes it is hard to know when to ask for help and when to try to stick it out on your own. It may also be hard for others to know when and how to help you. One man with Alzheimer's says, "A good caregiver doesn't enforce help. They offer, but then back off until I ask."

One of the first steps in accepting help is to acknowledge that some of your symptoms may interfere with your ability to accomplish certain tasks. Others might observe changes in your abilities that you may not notice. For example, you may think you are managing your bills and finances just fine, but a loved one notices that some of the bills are going unpaid or checks are not being recorded accurately in the checkbook. Or you may tell the doctor that you are taking certain medications, when in fact, you have run out of your prescribed pills and never refilled them at the pharmacy. It can be hard to accept that someone else is concerned about you when you don't think you have a problem.

The following signs indicate when accepting help may be practical, supportive, or necessary:

- You are repeatedly frustrated, angered, or discouraged when trying to complete a task. With help you could accomplish the task without wasting valuable energy.
- You are making mistakes that could be dangerous to yourself or others, such as errors in bank accounts, burning pots on the stove, or injuring yourself with a power tool. With assistance, you may be able to accomplish these activities safely.
- You are held back from doing one thing because you are unable to accomplish another. For example, you don't have company over for dinner because you can't make the whole meal yourself, or you no longer enjoy a hobby because you can't remember all of the steps. With assistance, you may be able to continue these activities.
- There is a time constraint requiring quicker action. For example, if you need to be out the door for a morning appointment, you may feel less

pressure and can be there on time if you allow your care partner to make breakfast for you.

Sometimes it is strategic to accept help. You may think you are losing control, but in fact you may be taking control of the situation by deciding to effectively partner with someone else. Bill Tuel has young-onset Alzheimer's and provides wise counsel, saying, "Don't be in denial about changes in yourself. Don't be ashamed to ask for help."[2]

Accepting Help Can Be a Gradual Process

Some people shun assistance because they don't want to feel supervised, or they find unwelcome help from others to be intrusive. Perhaps you feel demoralized by the way in which others take charge. Your loved ones may be frightened by concerns for your safety, or they may unintentionally be overbearing in their attempts to help you. One woman describes a painful encounter with her daughter who intercepted her attempts to cook:

> "A few days ago I was at the stove cooking chili...My daughter saw me cooking. Well, she came by and reached in front of me while I was at the stove...She reached right across my belly and turned off the stove as if I wasn't there...as if I was stupid...as if it didn't matter...It really hurt my feelings badly. She could have said, 'Mom you're the one who taught us to make that delicious chili, let's have some.' At this age, you hate to be ignored or chastised without words...We don't forget intentionally you know. It just happens to us. It could happen to you some day, but I hope not..."[3]

It is often easier to learn to accept help gradually and in small steps. Jean describes the process she went through when she began to have trouble managing her finances and people suggested she get help. She says:

"I fought during every single step in getting help. I'd argue, 'I don't need it. I don't need it yet. I don't want it now,' and so forth. Then eventually I think, 'I really do need help now,' and I get help. I don't know at what point this happens. It's something magical I guess. Yesterday it was out of the question and today it's, 'Ah, just do it. It won't hurt you. What's the problem?' Then I'm always glad I did do it after all. It's a slow process, I guess."[4]

Accepting help is not an all-or-nothing process. It may be difficult to accept assistance with some things, but easier with others. This may be confusing to you and your loved ones as you try to adapt to these adjustments, and it is not uncommon to have conflict about these issues.

"But If I Don't Use It, I May Lose It!"

You may be concerned that if you accept help from others, you will lose your remaining abilities. Lou Howes worries about this and writes:

"I know I would be better off by just letting other people do the things that I don't do well any more, but something in me says, 'Hang in there and keep on working with what I have left.'"[5]

Although it is important to make the most of your abilities and do as much as you can for yourself and others, it is also a positive coping skill to recognize when a little bit of help can go a long way. If you persevere alone to the point of extreme frustration or possible failure, you have accomplished little and are not improving your symptoms. Sometimes all it takes is a little prompt from someone else who finds a missing object, sets up the next step, or reminds you of that forgotten piece of information needed to accomplish your task. You can then proceed ahead and exercise your abilities more effectively and efficiently.

The Role of a Personal Assistant or Companion

If you always resist receiving assistance, you may be missing out on some added benefits. Some people hire a personal assistant and find that they actually have increased independence and the freedom to make choices about activities. One man employs an assistant for two days a week to drive him places and accompany him on activities. "Those are my favorite days of the week," he says. "We do what I want to do, go where I want to go, and I'm in charge. It's freedom!"

Personal assistants can come from various sources, including home healthcare agencies, your local Alzheimer's organization, senior center, friends, family members, or religious organizations. Consider the following circumstances when a personal assistant could be helpful. Keep in mind that your loved ones may notice some of these signs before you do:

- You are sleeping or watching television in excess and are not getting beneficial activity or exercise. A personal assistant can learn what kinds of activities you enjoy and help you spend your time more meaningfully.
- There are risks to your safety, such as forgetting to take medicine, or leaving the stove on. If you live alone or have a care partner who has obligations outside the home, a personal assistant can help to reduce the risk of an emergency or oversight.
- You have become lost, disoriented, or have fallen when taking a walk. A personal assistant can take walks with you or be on the lookout if you do not come back on time.
- Your care partner is burdened and needs help. Although you may not want help or feel you need it, agreeing to have an assistant help with meal preparation, housekeeping, transportation, or other tasks can relieve your loved one's stress.

Screen potential assistants for compatibility and reliability. You and your care partner can interview candidates, or you may already know someone who could be a good match. Jane says, "Now we have a lady in—a friend of mine. She lives with us now and she does most of the things…things that I find that I was having problems with, like cooking or commotions of people around me. She takes that off my shoulders and I'm at ease."[6]

By Accepting Help, You May Help Others

It may be difficult to come to terms with needing assistance, but learning to accept help when you need it is an essential strategy in coping effectively with Alzheimer's and can build bonds between people. Two people can often tackle a problem better than one. When you accept help, a task can be accomplished together, and you are better able to exercise your abilities.

In learning to accept help, you could be helping someone else in ways you may not even realize. A teenager, Holly Elizabeth Hedberg, writes in the Alzheimer's Foundation of America's publication, care*AD*vantage, a poignant story of how she learned the importance of accepting help from her father who had Alzheimer's:

> "Even while healthy, he never shunned assistance and never feared admitting a flaw. As his needs and flaws multiplied, his acceptance taught me to reach out to those around me for the support I needed…His complete humility and surrender to what he could not do alone showed me the folly of my own solitude. Since then, I have learned what I can handle, and, like my father, what I can't…I know that regardless of his forgotten things, my father knew how to live and now, by extension, so do I."[7]

Accepting and receiving help is a lifelong process for everyone. We may not always require someone to take full care of us, but we always need someone to care about us. In every step of the way, your lives and the lives of others can be enhanced by your ability to participate in this exchange.

Questions for Discussion

- Have you or a loved one observed times when you could benefit from assistance? If so, when?
- Have there been other times in your professional or personal life when you needed assistance from others? If so, what was that like?
- How do you respond to others when they offer to help you now? Are there better ways they can offer their assistance?
- What is there to lose by accepting help? What is there to gain?

Suggestions for Accepting Help

- Identify family members, friends, or professionals whose opinion you trust and respect. Work with these individuals to identify and write down circumstances in which you could benefit from some assistance.
- Share your feelings about accepting help so you can begin to work through any obstacles.
- When considering a personal assistant, find one who is familiar with Alzheimer's or willing to take classes, read, or learn about what you are experiencing. Evaluate shared interests as well as practical issues such as his or her ability to provide transportation.
- If your support group meets infrequently, try to find ways to get together socially with one or more of the group members in between meetings. This can help to build friendship and maximize the support and camaraderie you experience in your group meetings.
- It is important to consider your loved ones' feelings. If they are worried or overwhelmed, try to accept help to ease their stress. You might find that life runs more smoothly for everyone.

Chapter Seventeen

Finding Meaningful Activities

Everyone has varied amounts and types of activity throughout life, but for most people with Alzheimer's, memory loss and other symptoms begin to affect participation in previously enjoyed hobbies or interests. People cope with these changes in different ways. Millie recalls, "It was quite a blow when I realized I had Alzheimer's. I have a friend who has Alzheimer's, and the minute she found out she had it, she quit going anywhere because she said, 'Well, I just can't cope with it.' And I said, 'Well, that's silly because the only one who can change your situation is you!' So, I keep busy. If you're going to sit at home and say 'poor me,' that's exactly what is going to happen, and I don't let that happen to me."[1]

> *"There are lots of things which we can do to live active and useful lives with Alzheimer's."*

In this chapter we explore the importance of maintaining meaningful activity and offer some suggestions for ways to engage your interests and even develop new ones.

Overcoming Obstacles to Activity

Millie expresses a firm belief that in spite of Alzheimer's, she can influence the quality of her life and stay active. Others find it harder to get motivated. Some people feel they have adequate activity and social interaction, even though their care partner may observe that their loved one is unmotivated, does very little, and has limited social interactions. Because Alzheimer's symptoms can make it more difficult to do things, completing a few routine daily activities can seem like you've put in a full day's work. It is hard for others to see the effort an activity can require, and you may feel as if you are doing more than you actually are. Also, you might withdraw from previously enjoyed activities in an attempt to cope with or avoid symptoms. William Deutsch, a podiatrist who had to retire at age 56 due to the onset of Alzheimer's, says:

> "We become afraid to make mistakes, show our vulnerability, and thus, we cease to engage. This creates a vicious cycle of non-involvement and a gradual disappearance from whatever we consider to be a vital existence."[2]

Perhaps it is more difficult to do some previously enjoyed activities, or you need a boost from others to explore new ones. Finding and participating in meaningful activity may require some adjustments. One man says:

> "There are lots of people with early-stage Alzheimer's, and there are lots of things which we can do to live active and useful lives with Alzheimer's. I have lost some cognitive ability, but I have lots of ability left and I can work around the things that I can't do. That's one of the things that activity does; one learns how to work around a problem, just like learning how to avoid using a strained muscle. I'm so fortunate I was diagnosed early. It has given me the chance to do things that keep the beast at bay."[3]

The Importance of Socializing with Others

Research suggests that social interaction with others is an important part of maintaining your brain. Changes in memory or language abilities can make some social situations more challenging, but it is important to practice both expressing and listening to conversation. Social interactions that include activities are also stimulating. One man says, "My wife and I play cards with friends. The social part is important, and I also think that playing cards helps to stimulate my brain." It can also be enjoyable to socialize around a particular event. For example, going on an outing to a park, zoo, museum, movie, play, sporting event, or concert takes the emphasis off of verbal communication and allows for enjoyable companionship based on a shared experience.

Some people find that one-to-one interactions or small groups are easier to manage than larger groups. Regardless, it takes the pressure off of everyone if you let others know that you have Alzheimer's and are doing your best to stay active.

Participating in Specialized Programs

One way of maintaining social interaction can be through specialized community-based programs designed for people with early-stage Alzheimer's or a related disorder. Professional facilitators help people with mild symptoms capitalize on their strengths and abilities in a supportive environment in which everyone can be more at ease with one another. Although not all communities have these activities, there are a growing number of innovative programs that have been established across the United States and in many other countries to meet increasing needs.

Early-stage support groups are the most common type of program (see Chapter 15). However, other programs incorporate cultural outings in the community, mentally stimulating classes, volunteer work, creative arts, or activities that include family members. At MemoryWorks, a mentally stimulating program run by the New York City Chapter of the Alzheimer's Association, one participant says, "We can relax together and not feel like we have anything to prove here, so it gives us a chance to laugh a lot and forget about our dementia for awhile."[4] A participant of the Diablo Respite Center's women's club in Northern California gets together with other women who have early-stage Alzheimer's once a week. "The outings are a miracle...I get to go to wonderful places that I wouldn't be able to go by myself. This group gets us out into life and enlarges our lives. There are lots of diseases, and maybe this is not the worst."[5]

Many programs for people with early-stage Alzheimer's have been inspired by the requests or expressed needs of individuals and families and are sponsored by Alzheimer's organizations or research centers, adult day centers, religious groups, or other senior service agencies. Learn what may be available in your community, and speak up if there are no programs in your region.

Developing or Maintaining Enjoyable Hobbies

Some people enjoy hobbies throughout life, while others have never cultivated many interests outside of their work or their efforts to raise a family. Memory loss and other Alzheimer's symptoms may make it more challenging to engage in old or new hobbies, but it is important to make modifications if needed and explore possibilities for new interests.

Photography can be an enjoyable and stimulating hobby. One man says, "I take a lot of photographs, because then when I get the pictures developed, it's like I discover the thing I photographed all over again." A digital camera is an inexpensive option to explore. You can take as many pictures as you want and delete the ones you don't want to keep. Photos can also be downloaded onto a computer where you can view them as a slide show, or they can be printed and placed in photo albums. Choose a camera with a simple point-and-shoot function so you don't have to manage multiple settings. Taking photographs can help you pay attention to your environment, while reviewing your photos can help to prompt memory and provide hours of enjoyment.

Some people enjoy gardening for its creative, physical, and stress-reducing benefits. For others, working in the yard is somewhat of a chore, but it provides a productive activity and a contribution to home maintenance. Gardening often involves multiple steps that require memory and problem-solving skills, and it is important to do one task at a time. Some people benefit from having their own space in the garden where they can focus on one specific area and make it their own without fear of disrupting other home landscaping. Raised planter beds are a helpful addition to a garden, especially for growing vegetables or flowers. "I still like to garden, but I don't use all of the electric and gas-powered stuff that I used to," says one gardener with early-stage Alzheimer's. "It just moves too fast, so I use hand tools now. It's a lot more work!"[6]

You may enjoy sewing, woodworking, or a wide range of other hobbies. It is important to try to make necessary adaptations so you can continue to enjoy these activities. For example, if your sewing machine is becoming difficult to manage, have someone help you to set it up, so you can take the next step in your project, or shift to hand sewing with embroidery or other needlework. If power tools are no longer safe, switch to hand tools in your woodworking. These adaptations can be awkward at first, and you may be tempted to give up. But adapting is key to managing symptoms and continuing to stay active.

Physical exercise is also a very rewarding and meaningful activity for many people and can be incorporated into hobbies such as dancing or a variety of sports (see Chapter 19).

Reading Books and Watching Movies

Reading is a common activity. Perhaps you get the morning newspaper, subscribe to certain magazines, or are an avid fan of good novels. Although many people with early-stage Alzheimer's continue to enjoy reading, some people find that their memory loss or other symptoms interfere with this activity. There are ways to compensate for some of these challenges. (See Chapter 10 for a discussion on reading.)

Many people also enjoy watching movies. If memory loss begins to interfere with your ability to follow the plot of a movie, consider travelogues or documentaries that are focused on nature, travel scenery, or other action, such as sporting events. Musicals or comedies are enjoyable because they often emphasize lighter entertainment rather than complex stories. Also, repetition can enhance learning. If you have a home VCR or DVD player, consider buying some movies for home use. You can watch them as often as you like, and the plot and characters will become more familiar to you over time.

Recording Your Memories for Yourself and Others

Most people with Alzheimer's can clearly recount memories from the distant past, but yesterday's events are harder to recall. Even if your memory fails you for specific facts or details, it is likely that you can share many recollections, feelings, thoughts, and opinions with others. These reflections are an important part of your identity, and recording them in some way can create a meaningful legacy to others.

Some families use video cameras or tape recorders to record memories or discussions. You can speak directly into the recording equipment, or another person can ask you questions to prompt your replies. One woman says, "I've been working with my daughter to tape record my memories. It's hard for me to write these days, but I can sure talk! She asks the questions, and I do the talking, and we're having a lot of fun." Others make use of autobiography books available through bookstores or online to write down their reflections and personal history. Some books follow a simple question-and-answer format with ample lined space for writing the answer. Questions can vary from "What was one of your most memorable toys as a child?" to "What kinds of qualities do you look for in a friend?" and usually cover experiences about family, friends, education, work, and spiritual or philosophical beliefs. A family member or friend can ask you the question and then write down your reply. This provides an interactive activity that often sparks conversation.

Not all questions may appeal to you, or you may choose not to discuss some of the topics, but many of the questions prompt interesting reflections or memories that might otherwise never have been shared. Your book or other record of your thoughts will serve as a rich legacy of your life experience for your children or grandchildren. If you give these autobiographical journals a try, you might find that you have more of a memory than you think!

"Can I Still Travel?"

Travel is a meaningful activity for many people with Alzheimer's. "When I travel to a new place, it takes my mind off of all my worries," says Al. "I see new things and have different kinds of experiences than I do at home. I feel part of something bigger than my usual little world."

Alzheimer's may have little impact on your enjoyment of travel, but you might need to modify travel plans somewhat. Memory loss, as well as being out of your normal routines, increases your risk of losing things or becoming fatigued or disoriented. Many people with Alzheimer's continue to travel on longer vacations or tour foreign countries, but if such trips become too challenging, shorter weekend trips can be satisfying. You may enjoy a visit to a familiar destination, such as the home of family or close friends. Consider taking a few small trips to see how you adjust before embarking on a longer trip to an unfamiliar place.

When you plan for travel, the following tips may be helpful:

- Simplify your travel itinerary. See fewer places in greater detail so you have more time to get accustomed to new surroundings. Some people enjoy small cruise ships because the boat provides a consistent place for sleeping and eating with the opportunity to dock at different ports for day trips.
- Schedule "down time" during your trip when you are not on the go and can rest.
- Have identification with you at all times. Check with your local Alzheimer's organization for programs to enroll in, such as Medic-Alert/Safe Return, Comfort Zone, or Project Lifesaver International so you can receive assistance if you get lost or become separated from your group (see page 89).
- Bring a nightlight for your hotel bathroom so you can find it more easily in the dark.
- Pack lightly! Too many items and bags create more opportunities to lose things.

- Ask your doctor about a mild sleep aid to use if needed. Disrupted sleep and jet lag can increase confusion and disorientation. Do not use over-the-counter sleep aids without a doctor's approval, as they can increase confusion.
- Drink plenty of fluids. Travel (even in cool climates) can be dehydrating, resulting in worsened memory and confusion.
- Keep a simple diary or take photographs to help you recall each day's events and help you remember special details of your trip when you return home.
- Write postcards to friends and family. Ask them to keep them for you so you can have them as mementos upon your return home.
- Consider telling other travelers or tour guides that you have Alzheimer's or simply that you have memory loss. This may put everyone more at ease and allow others to help you if needed.

Enjoying and Participating in Holidays

Holidays can be joyful times filled with meaningful activity, but they can also put increased demands on your memory, concentration, and energy. Alzheimer's symptoms may make it harder to participate in traditions associated with these special events. It could be necessary to modify your customs or ask for assistance as needed. One woman says, "I used to write a note in each Christmas card, but that's too hard now. This year, I'm writing one letter to everyone that I'll make copies of and send out. I used to think they were less personal, but now I realize it's a lot easier!" A man who lives alone says, "I can't manage holiday shopping anymore, so I asked my daughter to go with me. We wrote a list and did it all in one day. Couldn't have done it without her."

If you enjoy participating in preparations for holidays or special occasions, focus on one or two tasks or adjust expectations as needed about your level of involvement. One man tells friends in his support group, "Sometimes I just sit back and watch. My wife likes things just so, and it used to bother me that I couldn't be more helpful. But now, I keep her company while she bustles around. She seems happier to just do things her way, and I'm less stressed."

Large gatherings of friends or family are common during holidays. While some people enjoy these festivities, others are overwhelmed by them. One woman says, "My husband and I decided that I do better in smaller groups rather than the huge family gathering. We're going to have a series of smaller events this year so we can spend special time with each section of our large family." Holiday preparations and celebrations can provide meaningful activity, but make room for quiet time to restore energy and reduce confusion. Perhaps one man's message offers the most significant piece of advice about holiday activity: "Keep it simple and focus on what's most important. Do something for someone less fortunate than you are. When you stop and think about it, there's a lot to be grateful for."[7]

Finding New Discoveries in Your Home and Community

Sometimes you don't have to travel far from home to find a new adventure or a stimulating activity. One man discussed a fun strategy for adding a little discovery to life:

> "Even though we've lived in our city for many years, my wife and I have decided to try to visit a new site in the area each week. It's good for both of us. It's amazing how many parks, little museums, exhibits, and odd off-the-beaten-path places there are to see. We're having a lot of fun."

Part of this couple's enjoyment is in reading the local paper each day to look for these new places or events. Although their discovery outing is usually once a week, each day they discuss new possibilities and enjoy making plans for their weekly event.

One woman is finding new discoveries in a previously routine activity. She says:

"I live with my daughter. I don't cook easily on my own anymore, but my daughter and I are cooking together now. We are trying new recipes we have never cooked before—simple things, but each dish has been new and like a little discovery."[8]

Pets Can Provide Enjoyable Companionship and Activity

Many people acknowledge the pleasures and benefits of having a pet. Pets can help reduce stress, improve mood, or prompt an owner to take a daily walk. Many describe their pet as a non-judgmental companion that won't blink an eye if they tell the same story twice!

Responsibility for a pet can also provide a satisfying feeling of value and purpose. Jan explains why she enjoys having her dog:

"Muffin doesn't care what kind of mood I'm in—she doesn't care if I remember her name. All she cares about is being my friend. I needed a little responsibility, but not too much, because there were so many responsibilities being taken away from me."[9]

If you do not have a pet and are considering getting one, it is important to take pet care requirements into consideration and to make sure that you have a care partner on board to assist when needed. Memory loss may limit your ability to remember feeding or grooming schedules. Although a pet can provide companionship, activity, and comfort, you or your care partner may be reluctant to take on added responsibilities, and these concerns must be carefully evaluated and respected. One man enjoys the company of a specially trained therapy dog who is brought to his house weekly through a community agency. He walks with the dog and looks forward to the visits, but does not have to worry about the responsibility of the dog's care.

Fish tanks or bird feeders can provide a calming influence for some people with Alzheimer's and may require less commitment. Harvey discusses the relaxing enjoyment of watching the birds from his back porch. He says, "We have a lot of bird feeders, and I can sit and watch those birds for hours. It's different every day. New birds come and go, and there are different ones in different seasons." He also enjoys the activity of filling the bird feeders, and he recently added a birdhouse to the backyard, hoping a bird will nest there.

Finding Ways to Help Others

Many people value the opportunity to be helpful to others and find meaningful activity through volunteer work. Ron says:

> "I do volunteer work now in a skilled nursing facility... I just want to hold a person's hand and talk to them a bit…People with Alzheimer's need to try to get everything they can out of life…I try to pretend a little bit. Like I happen to have this disease, but when I go to the nursing home, I don't have it. I'm only thinking of helping people. I'm not worried about me."[10]

You may be more apt to get involved if you include a family member or friend in the activity with you. Consider the following possibilities:

- Assist with mailings or other projects through your religious organization. One woman says, "I volunteer at my church with their monthly newsletter—lots of folding and stapling, but they appreciate it, and that makes me feel good."
- Help out at your community library, senior center, or other social service agency.
- Assist with serving meals at a shelter for the homeless.
- Read to children at day care centers.
- Assist community groups with beach or park clean ups.
- Collect toys for needy children during the holidays.
- Help with fundraising or advocacy work with your local Alzheimer's organization.

- Participate in Alzheimer's research.
- Volunteer your smile. One man says, "I like to try and make people smile. Just smiling at people throughout the day is a meaningful activity for me."

Taking Quiet Time to Rest and Restore

Everyone needs some time for peace and quiet. Make time for quiet activity that is engaging, but relaxing. Some people unwind by watching television or videos, or listening to music. Others enjoy quiet activities such as doing jigsaw or crossword puzzles, looking through a magazine, meditation or prayer, or an afternoon nap. Your loved ones may worry about you if they think you do not have enough activity or don't seem busy. But some people with Alzheimer's find that they are content with quiet time and are not bothered by having limited activity. It is important, however, that your care partner also has quiet and restful time as needed, so you might attend a program in the community, go out to lunch with a friend, or do something else that affords your loved one some time to rest.

Engaging activity is a meaningful component to each day and is essential to maximizing your strengths and stimulating your abilities. Your activity preferences need to be adjusted to your previous interests and your current circumstances, but it is never too late to try something new. Keep your mind open to new possibilities and you may discover some pleasant surprises.

Questions for Discussion

- What activities do you enjoy?
- Have you made any modifications or adjustments that have made it easier to do these activities?
- Have you begun any new activities as a result of Alzheimer's?
- Are there activities that you have given up? If so, why? How have you responded to these losses?

Suggestions for Finding and Participating in Meaningful Activity

- Make a list of the family members, friends, or professionals from community organizations or agencies that can help you identify possibilities for meaningful activity. You may not always like a suggestion, or you could be reluctant to try one, but it can help to keep an open mind and give it a try.
- Consider asking others to help you as needed in an activity rather than giving it up entirely.
- Don't be too hard on yourself if you fail at something or can't do it the way you want to. We succeed and fail at a variety of things all throughout life. If you have a history of being hard on yourself, be more forgiving of yourself and your current struggles. This is easier said than done, but very little is accomplished by punishing yourself with negative thoughts and judgments.
- Adjust your expectations of yourself. Members of a support group for people with Alzheimer's in Denver, Colorado, offer sage advice for staying active: "Do things that are fun and enjoyable, and surround yourself with active people. Keep trying. Know your limitations, but don't give up. Do the things that you can do."

Chapter Eighteen

Speaking Your Mind Through Advocacy

Around the world, people with Alzheimer's and related disorders are finding their voice as advocates for themselves, their families, and their communities. Some do this through involvement with their regional or national Alzheimer's organizations, while others make quieter but still powerful inroads toward greater understanding and care through sharing their thoughts, feelings, and needs with loved ones or friends. Maybe you are already motivated to be an advocate in the

> *Each time you speak out on behalf of yourself or others with Alzheimer's, you are being an advocate.*

Alzheimer's cause and are already involved in taking action. More likely, you may be thinking, "I can't do that." Perhaps you have never identified with the concept of advocacy, don't know what is involved, or avoid circumstances that may draw attention to you or place you in the spotlight. Advocacy takes many forms, however, and you may find that there are a number of ways to take small actions, speak your mind, or have a positive impact.

You Can Make a Difference

Each time you speak out on behalf of yourself or others with Alzheimer's, you are being an advocate. Maybe you decide to tell a family member what you need and act as an advocate for your own welfare. Perhaps you do or say something that changes the way someone else treats you or thinks about people with Alzheimer's.

Esther discusses responses she has received from friends when she tells them she has Alzheimer's: "They tell me, 'You don't look like you have Alzheimer's,' and I think they learn that you can look like you always have looked and still have Alzheimer's. It's not like I have a sign on my forehead now." By being honest with others about her diagnosis, she challenges common myths about people with Alzheimer's and becomes an advocate for greater awareness.

Support groups often provide a forum for participants with Alzheimer's to speak out or coordinate a message to others. Support group members have written group letters to Congress, created educational handouts for family and professionals, and participated in fundraising events together. Many people feel more motivated or confident when they participate in group efforts.

Others Can Learn from You

You have significant insights that can be of great value to students in the health-related and helping professions. People with Alzheimer's have been guest speakers in courses for social workers, medical students, psychologists, and other healthcare disciplines. Your testimony could provide one of the more meaningful ways that young professionals learn sensitivity and skills in caring for their clients or patients. Victor was interviewed by medical students at the University of California, San Diego, about his experience living with Alzheimer's. He says:

> "I felt that I could help them to realize what the problem is and become better doctors. My purpose was to tell them and

show them what a person with Alzheimer's is going through. I also say, 'Don't become a doctor if you don't care about people. You're hurting them and your profession. Go find something else to do. You must show that you care about people.' I want them to be sensitive to what human beings are. And the medical students were good. After the interview, the head doctor shook my hand and said he appreciated the interview and that I had done a good job."[1]

By participating in the education of young or even well-established professionals, you help to shape the quality of care that you and others may receive now and in the future. People with Alzheimer's also provide valuable contributions by educating themselves and others through support groups or other early-stage Alzheimer's forums. At the fifth annual Early-stage Alzheimer's Conference of the New Your City Chapter of the Alzheimer's Association, 83-year-old Mary Ladman gave the following opening remarks:

> "Coming together like this assures us that we are not alone. It gives us the courage to not lock ourselves away, which you notice we're not doing, but to continue to do the things we like to do. It gives people with the diagnosis of Alzheimer's a forum in which they can express themselves. It provides an opportunity to educate the public and to change the twisted perceptions that people have about those with Alzheimer's."[2]

A Call to Action

Sometimes advocacy work involves a larger mission that can have far-reaching impact. In their *Call to Action* petition to the Alzheimer's Association in 2005, Jenny Knauss, diagnosed with Alzheimer's, and her husband, Don Moyer, urged the Association leaders to have more direct communication and engagement with people living with symptoms. They advocated on behalf of people with Alzheimer's and wrote:

"We have a unique perspective and understanding of our own needs. Under the auspices of the Association, some of us have testified in public hearings at the national and state levels and have contributed to advocacy and educational programs, but we should have more active roles and greater collaboration with the national office and the chapters. Many of us have the time, energy, ability, and commitment to make a powerful difference in our own lives, the lives of others, and the mission of the Association."[3]

They proposed a series of action steps for the Association to take to begin greater inclusion, and numerous people with Alzheimer's, professionals, and family members signed their support to this petition.

In its Chicago offices in January 2006, the Alzheimer's Association convened its first meeting of an Advisory Group of People with Dementia from diverse geographic regions and ethnic backgrounds to help guide the organization in addressing the needs and challenges of people with Alzheimer's or a related disorder. Members with early-stage Alzheimer's now serve for one year and give feedback on current and potential activities of the association. They also advise on ways to increase the participation of people with Alzheimer's and related disorders in the leadership and services offered by the association and its chapters.

One action can lead to another and build momentum; one or two voices can quickly become a chorus. There are a growing number of ways for people to be engaged with their local Alzheimer's organizations, and your participation can make a rich contribution.

Educating Your Elected Officials

Each year the Alzheimer's Association mobilizes people with Alzheimer's, their families, and professionals to visit state and national congressional offices to advocate for increased awareness and funding of Alzheimer's research and services. Speakers with Alzheimer's provide some of the most compelling testimony to Congress. Dr. Bernard Reisman, a retired professor with Alzheimer's, spoke to the Bipartisan Congressional Task Force on Alzheimer's Disease:

> "While I am still able, I want to do whatever I can to speak out about Alzheimer's disease…We know that scientists are on the verge of finding ways to prevent and treat Alzheimer's and that the help and funding our government provides today may save future generations from this terrible thief that steals memories, disrupts careers, and affects millions of families. If the research can proceed fast enough, there may be something that will make a difference for me, but I pray that the discoveries will come in time for the next generation…We are in a race against time, and if we don't find the answers soon, Alzheimer's will be an epidemic."[4]

A growing number of people with early-stage Alzheimer's want to have a voice and be engaged in meaningful efforts to help the cause. One participant of a town hall meeting on Alzheimer's urged others to get involved: "We need to fight, so please keep your voices going and keep pushing and keep moving."[5]

An International Movement

Participation in advocacy work gives people with early-stage Alzheimer's an opportunity to take part in an international movement and make a difference. Alzheimer Disease International (ADI) is the umbrella organization for Alzheimer's associations and societies around the world. ADI has made important progress in recognizing and encouraging the contributions of people with Alzheimer's in its international work and now includes people with Alzheimer's and related disorders on its board of directors. Some individual countries are also working to be more inclusive of people with Alzheimer's in the planning and development of services and have developed focus groups or other forums through which to learn more about the needs of their citizens.

Lynda Hogg resides in Edinburgh, Scotland, and discusses the sense of purpose she derives from doing advocacy work. She writes writes in *Global Perspective—A Newsletter of Alzheimer's Disease International:*

> "I was introduced to the Scottish Dementia Working Group. This is a campaigning and awareness-raising group funded by Comic Relief and Alzheimer Scotland. It is run by and for people with dementia. Without a doubt this was a huge positive for me, as I became involved and the rest is history. I have given presentations, attended conferences, including an Alzheimer Europe conference in Portugal, been involved in a variety of other activities, and I am a former vice-chair of the group. This was my springboard into other things."[6]

With the advent of the Internet and more people reaching out via email, some people with Alzheimer's or a related disorder have organized online communities to provide forums for discussion, peer support, and advocacy, including Dementia Advocacy and Support Network International (DASNI) in the United States, and Dementia Matters out of Great Britain. The Web site of the Alzheimer's Association and a few other international Alzheimer's organizations include chat rooms for people with Alzheimer's and related disorders or offer others ways to connect with peers. Some regional and international conferences have break-out sessions for attendees who have symptoms, or they include scheduled times for them to meet for discussion and support. These opportunities remind participants that there is a global community that can ease feelings of isolation and open the door to the possibility of new relationships.

Taking Steps Toward Taking Action

Advocacy work can take whatever form suits you or your loved ones. It could be one minute you take to make a call, a morning's fundraising walk, an educational discussion with a friend, or a more ambitious trip to

Congress. Every effort counts.

The following suggestions are ways to be involved and make a difference:

- Share your experiences or concerns about Alzheimer's with others as a way of increasing awareness.
- Participate on local, state, or national committees. Call your local chapter of the Alzheimer's Association and tell them you want to be a volunteer or advocate.
- Help with fundraising activities for local and national Alzheimer's organizations.
- Provide your feedback as a person with early-stage symptoms to individuals or organizations that are developing services, writing educational materials, or providing care to people with Alzheimer's or a related disorder.
- Speak on panels or give talks at workshops, conferences, or other educational programs for families and professionals.
- Write a letter or an editorial for your local newspaper or Alzheimer's organization's newsletter to share your thoughts on living with symptoms.
- Volunteer to be interviewed by the press when they do stories about Alzheimer's.
- Write, call, or meet with politicians at the state or federal level to advocate for policies and funds aimed at improving the lives of families facing Alzheimer's.

You may not think of yourself as an advocate, or may not want to be drawn into the spotlight. But chances are you have important perspectives, messages, and ideas that could benefit others and help advance the cause. There are an increasing number of ways to speak your mind, and you might be surprised at the number of people who will listen. Leo Ferrari writes:

> "By sharing experiences of our uninvited encounter with Dr. Alzheimer, we can break through the barriers of silence and

loneliness. Let us not be ashamed of something that is not our fault. Rather, let us speak out proudly and loudly about it—even laugh—and realize that while we last, we too have our contributions to make to the rich tapestry of human life."[7]

Questions for Discussion

- Have you been involved in any kind of education or advocacy work concerning Alzheimer's? If so, what was your experience?
- Are you reluctant to participate in these kinds of activities? If so, why?
- What do you think are the most important things for the public to understand about Alzheimer's? What do your elected representatives need to know?

Suggestions for Making Advocacy or Educational Activities More Enjoyable

- Some people are concerned about the time commitment involved in doing advocacy work. If you would like to participate, realize that any amount of effort is worthwhile.
- Advocacy work can be more enjoyable when done with others. For example, join others in a local fundraising walk, or get your family together to write a letter to Congress.
- If you would rather not be public about your circumstances or your message, share your thoughts or opinions with a family member or professional who can make sure they are passed on to the appropriate individuals or organizations.
- For more information on advocacy opportunities contact: National Alzheimer's Association Advocacy and Public Policy Office at 202-393-7737 or www.alz.org/join_the_cause_advocacy.asp.

Chapter Nineteen

Boosting Your Physical and Mental Health Through Exercise

The benefits of exercise are well known. Regular exercise helps maintain a healthy heart, control weight, and preserve muscle strength. Exercise can also improve blood flow to your brain, elevate your mood, release tension, and maintain your flexibility and mobility. Many people with Alzheimer's find that physical exercise takes their mind off memory problems and provides a welcome, refreshing activity. Exciting research is also revealing ways that exercise may also be of specific benefit to the brains of people with Alzheimer's.

> *Research is revealing ways that exercise may be of specific benefit to the brains of people with Alzheimer's.*

If you are not mobile or have other physical limitations, keep reading this chapter. You can still participate in meaningful exercise programs that can be adapted to your needs.

Nourishing Your Brain with Oxygen

Your brain requires adequate oxygen in order to function. The brain makes up about 2 percent of your entire body weight, but consumes roughly 20 percent of the oxygen that you breathe. High blood pressure, heart disease, or elevated blood sugars (such as those attributed to diabetes) can all reduce blood flow and oxygen to the brain and worsen Alzheimer's symptoms. Exercise helps to prevent these other conditions, improve blood flow to the brain, increase oxygen levels, and build new connections between brain cells that may improve thinking abilities.

Researchers are also investigating ways in which exercise may help to reduce some of the shrinkage of the brain associated with Alzheimer's. Gradual shrinkage of brain volume is a part of the aging process, but the shrinkage is more significant in people with Alzheimer's and contributes to a decline in thinking and functional abilities. It is possible that people with early-stage Alzheimer's may be able to preserve their brain function and strengthen their thinking abilities for a longer period of time by exercising regularly. Many people do report that they think more clearly and feel more mentally alert after exercise.

Routine exercise can provide a pleasant form of both mental and sensory stimulation. One man says:

> "When I take my walk each day, I always see something new. I try to look at the gardens or see who is doing what to their house. I also like to see how many animals I can find—mostly cats and dogs, or maybe a squirrel, but it keeps me paying attention."

Exercise Can Improve Mood and Regulate Sleep

Many people who have Alzheimer's also experience symptoms of depression. The stress of living with memory loss and other symptoms, combined with changes in the brain chemistry, can result in feelings of sadness or apathy (disinterest in activity). Depression can also affect thinking and concentration and worsen some Alzheimer's symptoms. Doctors may prescribe an antidepressant, but it is well documented that routine exercise can also be a helpful remedy for depression. Exercise releases endorphines in the brain that contribute to a feeling of well-being. Many people report feeling brighter and in a better mood after physical exercise.

Alzheimer's can also affect sleep patterns. You may sleep too much during the day if you are depressed or do not have enough activity to keep you alert and physically active. Excess sleep during daytime hours can disrupt nighttime sleep patterns. Exercise can provide meaningful activity and help regulate nighttime sleep. Exercising too close to bedtime, however, may make it harder to fall asleep, so consider doing more vigorous exercise in the morning or afternoon.

Exercise Can Reduce Tension and Stress

Exercise can reduce feelings of irritability or agitation. These feelings can result from the frustrating daily encounters with memory loss and other symptoms. Everyone needs to let off some steam from time to time, and exercise is an excellent outlet for frustrations. Good physical exercise elevates the heart rate and seems to burn off tension and stress. Just as many feel more alert after exercise, others report the beneficial calming effects of physical activity. The focus on physical exercise can take the mind off worries and relax the thoughts. Enjoyable social activity can also reduce stress, and some people find that exercising with others gives the added benefit of social stimulation.

Maintaining Strength and Coordination

Some people with Alzheimer's become more sedentary, which can result in decreased muscle strength, bone density loss, and reduced flexibility. Maintaining strong muscles, balance, and coordination may help you function independently for a longer period of time and reduce your risk of injury from falls, sprains, or other accidents. Each year many thousands of seniors are admitted to hospitals and nursing homes after breaking a hip due to falling. The spatial and perceptual changes in vision that occur with Alzheimer's can increase your risk for falls, so it is wise to maintain balance abilities as well as good muscle and bone strength.

What Type and Amount of Exercise Is Best?

There are many forms of exercise, and you can find the one best suited to you. Walking and swimming are two of the safest and most popular methods, but you can also get your exercise by taking part in sports such as bowling, golfing, or tennis. Some get their exercise through enjoyable hobbies such as dancing or working in the yard. You can also check with your local senior center, athletic center, or gym for a variety of exercise classes. You may enjoy working with a trainer experienced in senior fitness who can help guide you through a stretching or weight-training routine. Weight training can help maintain both muscle tone and bone density. A growing number of people are also discovering the benefits of gentle forms of yoga or the Chinese practices of tai chi or qigong. These forms of focused exercise can help with strength, balance, and flexibility and can be adapted to people of all ages and physical abilities.

If You Are Physically Disabled

Exercise can be a rewarding and meaningful part of maintaining well-being for people with physical disabilities. If you have difficulty with movement or require a wheelchair, you may be able to benefit from exercise programs in your community specifically designed for people with physical disabilities. Check with your local senior center, community college, or university for programs or classes. Organizations devoted to Parkinson's disease can also be helpful resources for adaptive exercise programs.

Many exercise routines can be modified to respect your limitations while capitalizing on your existing strengths, and you may find that you are capable of doing more than you think. You can also consult your physician about the possible benefits of physical or occupational therapy. These therapists can work with you (often with the assistance of a care partner) to learn stretching routines or other exercises that can maximize your abilities, provide enjoyable activity, and help reduce your risk of injury.

Pay Attention to Safety When You Exercise

Sometimes people exercise to improve their well-being, only to end up injuring themselves in the process! Accidents can happen when you least expect it during any kind of routine activity, but exercise warrants particular caution and attention to safety. It is important to tailor a program to meet your specific needs, health condition, and body type. If you have a long history of exercising, you may be accustomed to a routine that works for you. If you are new to exercise or are starting a different type of activity, consult your physician before beginning your routine.

Any exercise should begin gradually and include gentle stretching before and after exercising so your muscles have a chance to warm up and cool down. Exercise in well-lit places, ideally with even surfaces. If you walk or jog, stick to routes with familiar terrain so you can avoid broken sidewalks or unexpected curbs. Walkers or hikers can also benefit from using a walking stick or hiking poles, available in outdoor and sporting goods stores, to assist with balance.

What if I Don't Like to Exercise or Can't Get Motivated?

If you do not enjoy physical exercise, at least try to gradually increase your daily physical activity. Consider the following simple opportunities for increasing your movement:

- Walk up a flight of stairs instead of taking an elevator.

- Sweep your sidewalk with a broom instead of an electric blower.
- Push your grandchild in a swing at the park.
- Throw a ball for your dog.
- Get up from your chair to get that cookie instead of placing the bag next to you.
- Dust your long-overlooked curio cabinet.
- Dance in your living room to your favorite music.
- Slowly pedal a stationary bike while you watch television.

Any movement is usually better than none. It does not have to be strenuous to be beneficial. But if you can gently get your body in motion a bit more throughout the day and periodically increase your heart rate, you may feel better and be motivated to increase your activity level.

If you pick a set time for exercise each day and develop a routine, you may be more apt to follow through. You can pair exercise with a reward for added incentive. Maybe you take a swim class with friends and then go out to lunch afterward, or, after walking at the mall, you do a little shopping. Many people also value having an exercise partner who provides companionship or encouragement. "Walks help me to get exercise, which I know is important," one woman says. "It also gives my husband and me time to talk."

Finally, remind yourself of the benefits of movement and exercise. The experience of Alzheimer's symptoms can be frustrating and discouraging, but for most people, there is very little physical decline associated with the early stages. Exercise can help to maintain or strengthen existing physical abilities while also having a positive impact in many other areas that affect your quality of life. If you follow sound safety precautions, exercise may be one of the more effective treatments for managing Alzheimer's.

Questions for Discussion

- Do you have an exercise routine? If so, are you happy with it?
- How can you increase your movement or physical activity throughout the day?

- If you do not enjoy exercise, what could make it more appealing?

Suggestions for Getting the Most Benefit from Exercise

- Consider exercise that engages you both physically and mentally. For example, yoga or tai chi practices usually include paying attention to your breathing; ballroom dancing requires that you remember specific steps; tennis may challenge your thinking when you try to keep score; walking with a partner or group may include conversation that stimulates your language abilities.
- Light snacks before exercise can be beneficial, but try not to eat a big meal right before exercising. Usually food intake an hour or so before exercise is optimal so that your body has time to digest and derive energy from the food.
- Consider varying your exercise and movement. Perhaps you walk one day, and do your stretching class the next. Maybe you worked in the yard yesterday, so you swim today.
- Involve people or pets in your physical activity. A child's request to toss a softball or a dog's need for a walk can provide good motivation to get moving.
- Don't be too hard on yourself if you don't exercise regularly. If it becomes a tedious physical chore that you dread, you become less motivated. Any increased movement can be beneficial, so create a personalized plan that works for you.
- Read, download, or order a free copy of *Exercise & Physical Activity: Your Everyday Guide from the National Institute on Aging* at www.nia.nih.gov/HealthInformation/Publications/ExerciseGuide through the National Institutes of Aging Information Center at 800-222-2225.

Chapter Twenty

The Benefits of Mental Stimulation

Many people have heard the saying, "use it or lose it." Although there are many well-known physical, emotional, social, and cognitive (thinking) benefits to keeping your mind active, when it comes to Alzheimer's, the saying is too simplistic. Although intellectual and social stimulation throughout life may help to reduce risk for Alzheimer's, many people who have maintained an active and engaged lifestyle still develop the disease. Moreover, increased mental stimulation cannot reverse significant memory loss or other Alzheimer's symptoms. There are ways, however, to maximize your existing skills, exercise your thinking abilities, and improve your quality of life through mentally stimulating activity. It is important to have realistic expectations about the benefits of these activities and to choose ones based on your interests.

> *Find the opportunities available in each day to exercise your brain and capitalize on your abilities.*

Making the Most of Your Abilities

Many of your previously enjoyed abilities may be challenged with the onset of Alzheimer's. It may take longer to do something, or the steps of an activity may require more concentration. However, research suggests that well-learned skills that you have practiced routinely during life may be retained the longest. You can continue to stimulate your thinking abilities by practicing what you are already good at. Sometimes this can be better achieved with a little guidance or assistance from someone else. For example, if you can no longer sew because you can't follow a pattern, partner with someone and do a project together. Break the task into small steps and take one step at a time. If you like to play golf, but can't keep track of your score, let your partner keep track while you focus on your swing. If you developed writing skills during your profession, use them now to record your thoughts, or start your autobiography. People who have become well versed in using a computer may find continued stimulation through surfing the Internet, writing a blog, or emailing with friends.

Some people give up on previously enjoyed activities if they can't do them with the skill or ease that they had once attained. While it may be more beneficial to modify activities rather than giving them up entirely, you will decide at what point a mentally stimulating activity becomes more irritating than engaging. Try to relax your expectations, give yourself more time, and focus on what you can still do.

Coping Strategies Can Stimulate Thinking

People with early-stage Alzheimer's often develop coping strategies that also stimulate thinking abilities. Many people use organization systems such as a calendar, notebook, or daily schedule. Each time you create and use such a system, you are doing a mentally engaging activity that exercises your thinking. One woman refers to her daily organizer as her "external brain," and her brain is very likely getting beneficial exercise each time she uses this tool. Some people develop photo albums of familiar faces they want to remember and routinely practice associating the picture with the correct name. Discussing facts, feelings, or memories about the people in the photos further engages your thinking and can help with retaining information.

There are likely many ways that you try to keep track of things each day, and the more you work toward developing effective strategies, the more you stimulate your thinking abilities.

The Importance of Paying Attention

If you are able to pay attention to and focus on an activity, you are more apt to benefit from its stimulating effects. We tend to better remember things that have captured our attention. Consider doing more of the kinds of activities that maintain your interest for a longer period of time. For example, if you like to do word puzzles, get a variety of puzzles that capture your interest. If you enjoy listening to music, attend more concerts and critique them with friends. Sometimes activities that are emotionally charged are more apt to capture the attention. Perhaps it's a good adventure movie or a reunion with a friend from the past that stimulates your emotions and engages your thinking. One man describes his nightly routine for charging up his attention and thinking: "Come 6 o'clock, I like to watch those commentators on the news stations. They all get worked up about politics and issues…My wife is amazed that I can remember what they are talking about enough to tell her later on."

You may also find that novel experiences that expose you to new people, places, or activities can be mentally stimulating. Anyone can get in a rut, so consider doing something you've never done before. Go to a new museum and take a guided tour through the exhibits, take a picnic to a different park than you normally visit, or enjoy a weekend trip to a new destination. Although repetition and routine are often effective methods for managing some tasks and maintaining practical skills, breaking out of the routine to enjoy new experiences can peak your attention and provide meaningful mental stimulation.

Social Interaction Is Mentally Stimulating

Anytime you engage in an activity that involves others, you are likely to be exercising your mind. Social interaction involves many areas of thinking, and it is important to find the types of interactions that are the most stimulating to you. Although some people do not identify with the concept of "support," they still find benefit in attending a support group where they can participate in engaging conversation. One man describes his weekly support group: "I don't think of it as a support group. It's more like a discussion group…We talk about things that are important to us."

Other participants may emphasize the learning that can occur when meeting with peers and appreciate the stimulation from social interaction. A participant of an eight-week educational support group for people with early-stage Alzheimer's says, "If you lost your memory 50 years ago, they put you off in a closet somewhere. They never had classes like this."[1]

Although still rare, a growing number of community programs designed for people with early-stage Alzheimer's are beginning to include group cognitive stimulation activities that incorporate trivia, puzzles, words games, and other opportunities for challenging the brain. These activities, combined with the group interaction, can give the brain an enjoyable workout.

Some people also appreciate social interaction that stimulates long-term memories. Alzheimer's mostly affects your short-term memory, so many long-term memories are intact. It can be enjoyable to reflect on positive memories in your life and to share them with others. Perhaps you have an alumni group, a veterans club, or a friend with whom you share a rich history. Social interactions that prompt reminiscence may stimulate long-term memory, while the conversation can exercise language, attention, and listening abilities.

The Business of Brain Fitness

The last decade has witnessed a booming market in programs and products aimed at brain fitness. Marketing is generally directed to aging consumers who want to exercise their brains in the hopes of preventing Alzheimer's. But what if you have already been diagnosed? A growing number of studies are examining whether people with Alzheimer's can benefit from structured "cognitive training" programs that aim to improve memory and other areas of thinking. So far these studies have revealed limited benefits to these programs. Although it may be possible to improve on a particular puzzle or drill that you practice repeatedly, this improvement may have little benefit to daily functioning and other activities. For example, memorizing a list of words in a brain exercise will not necessarily improve your ability to remember a neighbor's name, and finding the correct words to complete a crossword puzzle won't prevent you from losing your words during a conversation. Structured brain fitness programs can also be time-intensive and require discipline or ongoing daily practice in order to achieve limited outcomes.

If brain fitness programs and products engage your attention and provide a pleasant challenge, then you are likely providing meaningful stimulation to your brain. If, however, you are frustrated, bored, or demoralized by these programs, there is no evidence that hammering away at them day after day will provide your mind or mood much benefit. There may be many other ways to exercise your thinking abilities that could provide more meaningful value.

The Max Planck Institute for Human Development in Germany and the Stanford Center on Longevity at Stanford University in California convened a group of expert scientists to study the evidence behind the claims of various brain fitness programs marketed to consumers. After significant review, this esteemed group of scientists concluded:

> "Before settling on a particular method and investing time and sometimes money in a particular product, consumers need to consider hidden costs beyond dollars and cents. Every hour spent doing solo software drills is an hour not spent hiking, learning Italian, making a new recipe, or playing with your grandchildren. Other avenues for cognitive enhancement, such as participating in your community and exploring your passions, may also stimulate your mind while producing socially meaningful outcomes."[2]

These scientists caution consumers to be leery of any product that claims to cure or prevent Alzheimer's, since there is currently no evidence to justify such claims.

Do More of What You Enjoy

The bottom line for selecting ways to benefit from mental stimulation is to find out what sparks your attention, capitalizes on your abilities, might involve some social interaction, and results in a satisfying or enjoyable experience. Then do more of these things! If you want workbooks or manuals, this may seem like overly simplistic advice, and there is certainly no harm in pursuing more structured brain stimulation programs. For many people, however, the key to staying mentally stimulated is to find the opportunities available in each day to exercise your brain and capitalize on your abilities.

When asked, "What do you do to keep your mind stimulated?" people with early-stage Alzheimer's gave the following replies that illustrate the many paths to achieving this goal:

- Every week I have a *Newsweek* magazine that I listen to through Books on Tape. I also get *Reader's Digest* through the same program.
- If I feel troubled, I get out my watercolors and paint until the demons are gone. Then I write at the bottom what I was feeling.
- I am in a group that translates Greek poetry. It's taking me longer than it used to, but I still enjoy it very much.
- I am volunteering at the Adult Literacy Program. I can be around people and also give something back to the community.
- I like to go to cultural events, like concerts.
- I do crossword puzzles in the newspaper and I take notes every week at our Alzheimer's support group so we have a record of what we talk about.
- I read a lot—mostly war mysteries. My wife comes up with a lot of things for me to do!
- I can still take charge of the checkbook. That certainly keeps my mind challenged.
- My husband is interested in theater, so we go to the theater a lot.

- I don't think I do enough to keep my mind active. I probably should be doing more!

Questions for Discussion

- How do you keep you mind stimulated?
- Are there activities you once enjoyed that you have given up on that you could continue to do with assistance?
- Have you tried any brain fitness programs? If so, what was your experience?

Suggestions for Staying Mentally Stimulated

- Ask yourself each morning what you plan to do during the day to stimulate your mind. Write down your thoughts and try to do at least one of those intended activities that day.
- Try to do a variety of activities that engage various senses and areas of thinking.
- Explore whether your local Alzheimer's organizations have any mentally stimulating activities in your community for people with early-stage Alzheimer's.
- It is alright to stop doing any activity that produces more frustration than fulfillment. Attempts at mental stimulation that provoke excess stress are not productive, and you have a right to pick and choose what is most meaningful for you.

Chapter Twenty-One

Food for Thought:
The Value of Good Nutrition

Your food choices have significant impact on your physical and emotional health, and certain nutrients and diets are being investigated for the ways in which they may be able reduce the risk of developing Alzheimer's. The Mediterranean Diet has received the most attention for its beneficial emphasis on fresh fruits and vegetables, beans, fish, olive oil, moderate wine intake, and limited dairy and red meat consumption. But what if you already have Alzheimer's? Can diet have an effect on symptoms or their progression? There is no specific diet or food that can cure Alzheimer's, but growing evidence suggests that what you eat impacts your brain health. Good nutrition can also prevent other medical conditions that can worsen Alzheimer's symptoms.

> *Good nutrition can prevent other medical conditions that can worsen Alzheimer's symptoms.*

What's Good for the Heart is Good for the Brain

Much research suggests that cardiovascular health is linked to brain health. There may be a relationship between the high cholesterol associated

---

with heart disease and the beta amyloid protein involved in Alzheimer's. It is wise to keep your cholesterol within the limits advised by your doctor and adhere to a diet, such as the Mediterranean Diet, that also promotes heart health. Cardiovascular disease and incidents of large or even small strokes (called transient ischemic attacks, or TIAs) can complicate Alzheimer's and worsen symptoms. Some studies suggest that people who take specific cholesterol-lowering drugs (statins) get Alzheimer's at a lower rate than the general population, but research into statins has been inconsistent in showing benefit for treating Alzheimer's once symptoms have developed.

Your heart pumps blood to your brain and impacts the amount of oxygen that is delivered to your brain cells. It is important to maintain a healthy heart so your brain gets the nutrients it needs.

Protecting Brain Cells with Antioxidants and Omega Fatty Acids

Much research has explored the possible benefits of antioxidants in maintaining brain health. Antioxidants help to eliminate *free radicals* from the body. Free radicals are products that are released from normal cells but can cause damage to the cell, or accumulate in the brain plaques associated with Alzheimer's. Antioxidants may also help to reduce inflammation in the brain. Foods that are particularly rich in antioxidants include dark-green, leafy vegetables such as broccoli, spinach, and kale, as well as various berries, particularly blueberries. Tumeric, a spice common in Indian curries, contains a compound called curcumin that is also a powerful antioxidant, and recipes containing tumeric may be a beneficial addition to the diet.

Certain beverages, particularly pomegranate juice, are rich in resveratrol, a naturally occurring substance that may help to break down accumulations of the beta amyloid protein associated with Alzheimer plaques. Resveratrol is also an antioxidant, as is green tea.

Omega-3 fatty acids, particularly DHA, may also be helpful to both the heart and the brain due to their anti-inflammatory properties. Foods rich in omega-3 fatty acids include eggs, organ meats, spinach, flaxseed oil, and walnuts. One of the greatest sources of DHA is fish, but some worry about toxic levels of mercury found in fish. Some of the safest fish sources of DHA include wild salmon (not farmed), light tuna (not albacore), sardines, and shrimp. Although foods rich in DHA and DHA supplements have not been shown to improve Alzheimer's symptoms, they are certainly healthy food choices that may have subtle but important benefits to brain health.

The Effects of Alcohol on Alzheimer's Symptoms

Alcohol consumption affects each person differently. Excessive alcohol consumption over time kills brain cells and can lead to a dementia called Wernicke-Korsakoff Syndome. Although a history of mild alcohol intake may actually help to prevent Alzheimer's, many physicians recommend that people who do develop Alzheimer's should limit or eliminate their alcohol intake. Alcohol can temporarily worsen Alzheimer's symptoms by impairing concentration, memory, speech, problem solving, and judgment, as well as physical coordination and balance. Alcohol intake can also increase irritability, contribute to depression and difficulties with sleep, and interact dangerously with certain medications.

Consult with your physician about alcohol consumption. Any recommendations may depend on your alcohol use history, the medications you are taking, and the impact of alcohol on your Alzheimer's symptoms. If your physician recommends abstaining from alcohol, consider switching to non-alcoholic beer or wine that is available in most supermarkets.

Can I Still Have My Morning Cup of Coffee?

Alzheimer's does not have to interfere with your enjoyment of coffee unless your doctor advises otherwise. If you have always been a coffee drinker or enjoyed your cup of black tea, you have likely adapted to the caffeine in these beverages and may not need to alter your patterns. Indeed, some people find that their mood and thinking is somewhat improved by the temporary boost of a little caffeine. Keep in mind, however, that caffeine can elevate your heart rate and may increase irritability, anxiety, or insomnia in some people with Alzheimer's. Sodas and chocolate also contain caffeine. Due to memory loss, it could be easy to lose track of caffeine intake throughout the day, so some caution is warranted.

Maintaining Healthy Weight and Eating Habits

It is not uncommon for people with Alzheimer's to lose weight. Not all weight loss is cause for concern, and it may actually be welcome. However, persistent unintentional weight loss can weaken your body and lead to fatigue, loss of overall strength, increased confusion, and a compromised immune system.

Weight loss can occur due to:

- Nausea or gastrointestinal side-effects from Alzheimer's medications.
- Decreased sense of smell and taste that affects enjoyment of food.
- Forgetting to eat.
- Feelings of sadness or depression that reduce appetite.
- Ill-fitting dentures or other uncomfortable dental or mouth conditions.
- Reduced calorie intake due to difficulty preparing food.

If you used to enjoy food and now have less interest, it is important that you be medically evaluated for depression or any discomfort in your mouth that may be interfering with your enjoyment of eating. Although a loss of smell and the resulting reduction in taste is common with Alzheimer's, certain medications can also interfere with taste. You may begin to add more salt, sugar, or strong-tasting condiments to your food to enhance flavor and offset diminished taste. While this may be safe for some, this could be dangerous if you have other particular health concerns, such as diabetes or high blood pressure.

Weight gain is less common in people with Alzheimer's but can be due to:

- Poor eating habits.
- Medications that may increase weight.

- Withdrawing from previously enjoyed activities and becoming more sedentary.
- Eating more out of boredom.

Memory loss can make it hard to remember if you have eaten, so you may go back for more! Others just eat to have a pleasant activity. One man says, "I like to eat a lot! No matter how bad my memory is, I still enjoy a good meal." Many people with Alzheimer's also find they have more of a sweet tooth and may be drawn to cookies, candies, and ice cream. An occasional treat may be harmless. However, excess sweets can dull your appetite for more nourishing food, throw blood sugar levels out of balance, and contribute to significant shifts in mood or energy.

Making the Most of Meals

You might eat three meals each day, or perhaps you prefer to snack lightly throughout the day. Routines surrounding food are personal and are not necessarily affected by Alzheimer's. However, you may enjoy your meals more if you eat in a quiet, pleasant environment with few distractions. If you go to restaurants, consider ones with limited background music or other stimulus. Seek a booth or table away from the sounds and commotion of the kitchen. When weather allows, outside seating in a quiet courtyard or other patio can be preferable. You may alter some of your routines by going to restaurants earlier for meals before the crowds arrive. One person discusses the importance of letting friends and family know your needs:

> "I have a difficult time with noise. Going out to dinner causes problems for me because restaurants are so loud, so I have to tell my friends that. They're still wanting to go to lunch with me, but at 11:15 instead of noon. For me it's a big change, but my friends would never think about it so we have to help educate our family and our communities as to what we can and cannot deal with."[1]

Although uncommon, some people with early-stage Alzheimer's have visuospatial problems (problems with perception or judging where objects are in relation to things around them) that can make it challenging to eat off patterned china. It may be hard to distinguish the food from the plate. Likewise, white mashed potatoes may be hard to detect against a white dish. If you have visuospatial problems, try to eat on simply designed surfaces that provide good contrast against your food.

Mealtime can provide an enjoyable chance to socialize with others. Food is a basis for many celebrations, holidays, or opportunities for conversation among friends and family and can continue to be a meaningful part of your quality of life. Maintaining good nutrition and healthy eating habits is beneficial to both your physical and emotional health and is an essential ingredient in living your best with Alzheimer's.

Questions for Discussion

- Have you noticed any changes in your eating habits? If so, what are they?
- Have you lost or gained considerable weight recently? Is so, have you discussed this with your doctor?
- What makes mealtimes enjoyable for you? Are there times when they are less pleasant?

Suggestions for Maintaining Good Nutrition

- Some people find that snacking on small meals is easier and more satisfying than eating three big meals.
- Keep healthy snacks available, including fresh fruit, crackers and cheese, yogurt, nuts, and any other kind of satisfying finger food that does not require much preparation.
- Due to a reduced sense of smell, some people with Alzheimer's are at risk of unintentionally eating spoiled food. Date containers of leftovers before refrigerating. Do not keep leftovers for more than a few days,

and be sure to check the refrigerator regularly for spoiled food.

- Stay hydrated! Drink plenty of water and juice unless otherwise indicated by your doctor. Dehydration can result in confusion or urinary tract infections that can complicate Alzheimer's symptoms.

- Talk with your doctor to make sure that your levels of vitamin B12, calcium, iron, and other necessary nutrients are being adequately supplied by your diet. Deficiency in critical nutrients can compromise your physical and mental health.

Chapter Twenty-Two

Maintaining Hope and a Sense of Humor

Is this the first chapter you sought when you opened this book? If so, you have your priorities in order! And if you have read everything to this point, you may now wonder why you didn't start here. Hope and humor are not the first words that come to mind when you think of Alzheimer's, but they are two of the most important ones. The ability to laugh and to find promise in the future is an enduring and powerful gift to be reopened and savored over and over again. Read this chapter as many times as you like, because messages of hope and humor certainly bear repeating.

> *"It's OK to have a sense of humor. People with Alzheimer's do some pretty funny things!"*

The Gift of Humor

Many people with Alzheimer's and their loved ones discuss the benefits of finding humor in everyday life. Laughter can reduce stress. The act of laughing releases endorphins (a naturally occurring brain chemical) that foster a sense of well-being and relaxation. Endorphins are also released during exercise. A good belly laugh is a form of gentle exercise as it engages your chest, abdominal, and facial muscles and temporarily increases your heart rate and blood pressure. When the laughter subsides, your heart rate and blood pressure can actually drop lower than they were before you were laughing, resulting in a more peaceful feeling.

Laughter among family members and friends can brighten dark moments and promote more relaxed and encouraging feelings. One woman with Alzheimer's says, "It's OK to have a sense of humor. People with Alzheimer's do some pretty funny things!" Members of a support group for people with Alzheimer's in the San Francisco Bay Area in California advise their family members: "Have a sense of humor! It helps us to lighten up about things we may have trouble with."[1] The ability to laugh at one's circumstances can provide welcome relief. Al says, "Sometimes I feel like a big kid. Every day is a new day with new discoveries because I can't remember anything I've already discovered! I laugh about it and that keeps me young at heart."

Humor can often form a bond between people and lift everyone's spirits. Jay, a retired Air Force pilot, was diagnosed with Alzheimer's in his early 50s. He relies on a wry sense of humor to cope. One day while watching children enjoy an Easter egg hunt, he leaned over and told his neighbor, "Now that I have Alzheimer's, I can hide my own Easter eggs!" Humor can also help to put others at ease. Another man with early-stage Alzheimer's states, "I know how uncomfortable I would feel if I knew one of my friends had Alzheimer's...I decided to defuse the situation. If they ask me how I am feeling, I say 'Great! I haven't lost my keys all day!'"[2]

People with Alzheimer's often share a robust sense of humor with one another. During a support group meeting in California, one woman starts to say, "I think I may have already shared this story...," but is interrupted by another participant who says with a raucous laugh, "Hey, tell us again! Do you really think we've remembered it?" A sense of humor can also go a long way in helping you make it through the day-to-day challenges of Alzheimer's. Bea describes the problems she has with all of the steps involved in getting dressed every morning. She relies on her husband for assistance, but since he has had a stroke, she recognizes that it can be a difficult process for them both. She says, "I don't know what to do, and he doesn't know what to do, so neither of us does anything. Maybe I should just join a nudist colony!"

Members of the Alzheimer's Association Rocky Mountain Chapter Early-stage Support Group in Colorado know that humor is good medicine for Alzheimer's and have identified a number of ways that humor enriches their lives. They note that it relieves tension and stress, gives you energy, lifts your mood, helps manageembarrassing moments, can be a shared activity with others, and is contagious. Although humor can be therapeutic, these support group members also advise their family members and others to be sensitive about its use. They suggest that humor is not helpful if it is making fun of someone in a hurtful manner; if it leaves someone feeling left out; or when it's hard to understand. They caution that the use of humor could stifle other more serious feelings that need to be expressed.[3]

Feeling and Maintaining Hope

You may wonder where to find hope in the experience of Alzheimer's, but it lives in more places than you might imagine. It is not always easy to feel hopeful under challenging circumstances, but people with Alzheimer's discuss many different ways they continue to feel encouraged about their lives.

In his public address to the Alzheimer's Association of South Australia, Philip Alderton told his audience:

> "We may not be able to change the end result, but our journey there could well be determined by our actions and mental attitude. My feelings are that there is always hope. Wherever there is life, there is hope, however slender that may appear at times."[4]

Gloria challenges the philosopher Rene Decarte's famous words, "I think, therefore I am," and replaces them with, "I hope, therefore I am." Since the onset of Alzheimer's, she says she doesn't think as clearly, but she refuses to let that define who she is. In her powerful statement, she has decided that her self-esteem and sense of identity are based more importantly on her ability to be hopeful and to look for the opportunities in each day. Jim also recognizes the new possibilities each morning brings and remarks, "Waking up each day gives me hope!"

Although any disability can be discouraging, it is important to stay involved in life—to maintain activity that keeps you stimulated and challenged. John states, "Keeping active, getting around, and doing things gives me hope because if I don't keep doing things, I mope." A positive attitude is also essential. Another man says, "Looking on the positive side of things gives me hope. The negative doesn't do any good."

Thaddeus Raushi defies prevailing beliefs about Alzheimer's and offers a powerful message of hope. He writes:

> "I'd like to suggest that there are Alzheimer's survivors. For me, surviving is both attitude and action. It means that even while knowing that I have this disease, I can still go on with life always doing the best I can with what I have at any given point. This is the attitude of seeing life worth living. This is also the action of moving ahead with doing whatever is quality living at that moment…As my wife and I move forward together, we want to be able to know when to deal with the disease's issues and when to put them on the shelf. We want to both take the changes and behaviors seriously and at the same time be able to have a sense of humor about them…We want to remain believing that we are, at any time in our relationship and decision making, doing the best we can with what we have."[5]

Hope is also nurtured through the encouragement you receive from others who understand your challenges. Participants in Alzheimer's support groups frequently speak about the value of coaching one another along during the tough times. One participant says, "People coming together, and having everyone hoping together and thinking this way as a group, helps a lot." For those who do not participate in a support group, Rene speaks to another invaluable source of support, "I get hope from my grandkids and my family." If you have limited family relationships, it can be very comforting to establish a sense of extended community—a network of even one or two significant people who you know will see you through the ups and downs, and with whom you can share your hopes and your fears. True communication and understanding between people is one of the most powerful ingredients in a recipe for hope.

People with Alzheimer's and their families frequently seek information about research or clinical trials aimed at treating symptoms or preventing progression. Advances in science can provide much hope, and participation in research can be an effective way of coping with feelings and being proactive (see Chapter 30). One man provides the following sound advice: "We are still looking for the wonderful piece of medication that will provide a cure, but in the meantime we need to learn some new songs and some new jokes!"[6]

The Solace of Spiritual Faith and Practice

Some people with Alzheimer's have a longstanding spiritual faith or practice that helps them cope. One woman discusses how she draws on her religious beliefs to find a reason or meaning in having Alzheimer's. She says:

> "I pray a lot for God to give me strength and for my husband to have strength to go through this. If it's meant to be, then it's meant to be. As everyone would do, I wondered, 'Why me?' But then I realize God knows what he's doing and he'll take care of me. I have to trust God."[7]

Spirituality or a religious practice can provide hope, strength, guidance, or something to hold onto during tough times. In the video, *Alzheimer's Disease: Voices from the Journey*, produced by the Mayo clinic, Rick talks about the comfort derived from his faith: "You've got to have something to hold onto and my faith in God is something to hold onto."[8]

Relationships between people with Alzheimer's and their loved ones may also be enhanced by the hope or solace found in mutual spiritual beliefs or practices. Kathleen reflects on the changes in daily life with her husband Bill, who has Alzheimer's. She states:

> "We'll go on a walk and he'll be so excited about a rabbit or some other animal we may see. On one of our walks, there were a lot of snails on the path, and people crushed them as they walked. Bill was stopping and picking up the large ones and throwing them in the shrubs, trying to save their lives. These are the precepts of Buddhism—the reverence for life—that have stuck with me, and with Bill, too. Before Alzheimer's, he probably wouldn't have stopped; there was always something else going on. So, you just slow down and appreciate the small things."[9]

For some, their spiritual practice may undergo changes due to Alzheimer's symptoms. Gail says, "The first time I couldn't say the Hail Mary I cried. That is when I began meditating. Religion is just a word meaning 'to bond us to something.' Going to church is not the only way. Do what suits you."[10]

One man derives his hope, strength, and inspiration from the profound beauty of nature. He says:

> "It would be much easier if I clung to any religion. I'm sure this would be an advantage, but my mind is not going to go along with that. Religion is not what I need to get through Alzheimer's. I used to get away from the office once in awhile and go up alone in the mountains…I always cried. It's so beautiful! That is my religion. It's the biggest piece of religion that I know."[11]

Can Something Good Come from Alzheimer's?

It may be hard to imagine that any part of your life could change for the better as a result of Alzheimer's. However, finding and acknowledging positive outcomes from challenging or unwanted situations can greatly improve quality of life for you and your loved ones. Perhaps something encouraging has happened in your relationships with others, in adjustments you have made in your daily routines, or in insights you have gained into yourself. E.L.Gorman writes:

> "Yes, having Alzheimer's has changed my life; it has made me appreciate life more. I no longer take things for granted. I realize that time is precious and not to be wasted on negative emotions like anger, revenge, and hatred. I have learned the power of forgiveness. My grandfather used to tell me, 'Kill them with kindness.' I now understand what he meant."[12]

Participants with Alzheimer's at the Shiley-Marcos Alzheimer's Disease Research Center in San Diego were asked, "Has anything good come out of having Alzheimer's?" Here are some of their answers:

- I've learned to slow down a bit and find something to enjoy in each day.
- I spend more time with my grandkids now and my own kids say they have more time with me now than they've ever had before.
- I'm learning to be more patient with myself and others. Or I'm trying, at least.
- We got a dog so I would have some company, and that dog is the best thing that has happened to me in a long time!
- Yes, my wife and I will have an argument, and not long after, I've forgotten about it!
- I've met some great people in my support group. I didn't choose to get Alzheimer's, but I've found some new friends.
- I'm more flexible now. I know I can't always call the shots.
- I've become more physically active. Long walks help me stay strong and keep my mind off of my problems.
- I've realized that I think people are basically good. I don't like to ask for help, but when people find out my problem, they are usually kind and don't treat me strangely, so that's something good.[13]

Your life will continue to reveal many opportunities to experience the sustaining benefits of both hope and humor. Keep an eye and ear out for the possibilities, and never miss out on a chance to laugh, give thanks, and feel the promise inherent in each day.

Questions for Discussion

- Do you and your loved ones share a sense of humor? Is it helpful? Is it ever hurtful?
- What gives you a feeling of hope?
- Do you have a spiritual faith or practice that helps you cope? Have your beliefs been affected by the onset of Alzheimer's? If so, how?
- Has anything good come out of Alzheimer's for you or your loved ones?

Suggestions for Maintaining Hope and a Sense of Humor

- Rent funny movies or watch your favorite comedies. Clip out comics from the daily newspaper that make you laugh and put them in a scrapbook so you can reread them.
- Make a list of the people, situations, thoughts, or things that give you hope.
- Keep a journal of inspiring events that happen during the day. Review these experiences with your care partner so you can record these thoughts together.
- If your spiritual faith or practice has been challenged by the onset of Alzheimer's, consider talking about these concerns with your religious clergy or spiritual advisor.

Chapter Twenty-Three

Taking Care of Your Care Partner

The words caregiver, or care partner are frequently used in discussions of Alzheimer's to describe a person who gives emotional or physical care to another and provides assistance with routine daily activities. Although the emphasis is usually on how others give care to you, it is important to consider how you can be a partner in this process and reciprocate. Your memory loss and other symptoms will mean that you need more assistance from family, friends, or others, but there are many ways that you can extend care in return. When you help the people who are trying to help you, a sense of teamwork can develop that allows you to more effectively face challenges together.

> *Care partners need their own time for self-care that is both relaxing and restoring.*

As you read this chapter, think about the ways that you can express care for the people who are trying to care for you and how you can be a partner in this exchange.

Understanding Your Care Partner's Feelings

Your loved ones are going through their own feelings and life changes as a result of Alzheimer's. Although you may identify with some of the emotions, many people with Alzheimer's have limited awareness of their care partner's experiences. Your loved ones may need support with their own feelings, including:

Sadness

Just as you may grieve certain losses, your loved ones grieve over the effects of Alzheimer's on their own lives, too. Caregiver support group members write, "We have all mourned the loss of what used to be and what won't be in the future." Your loved ones are also at risk of becoming discouraged or depressed and will need to watch their own mood carefully.

Fear or Anxiety

It is common for care partners to have their own fears about Alzheimer's and how they will manage. One wife recalls her response to her husband's diagnosis: "I wondered how I would cope. My husband was always in charge. Now I would have to be responsible for everything." Your loved ones will need to learn new skills and access available resources to help ease their fears.

Anger

Care partners can feel angry about Alzheimer's. It was not part of the plan, and some feel ill-equipped to rise to the occasion. "We are not all heroes," writes Carol Levine. "We are not all going to live up to the standards of greatness. We are not all going to have the necessary resources—financial, family, and other—that will let us be perfect."[1] Care partners may be challenged to adjust expectations for themselves and their lives so they can regroup and rally the necessary support to manage challenges effectively.

Impatience

Memory loss and other Alzheimer's symptoms can be frustrating for other people. This is not your fault. However, it is important to realize that your loved ones are making adjustments to these problems, too. Lorna Drew's husband has Alzheimer's, and she writes, "I didn't realize that I was so short tempered. That realization has taught me something, and I am in the process of not only trying to learn patience, but also of forgiving myself when I fail."[2]

Feeling Stressed or Overwhelmed

Loved ones are assuming new roles and responsibilities while also trying to make sense of your feelings and experiences. Jim imagines how hard it is for his wife: "The role of a caregiver? I wouldn't take it at any price. I can be a real pain! My wife has to be a caregiver and a psychiatrist at the same time." A wife appreciates when her husband with Alzheimer's recognizes her feelings and expresses concern. "He notices my stress, and that helps a lot."

It can be difficult to acknowledge the effects of Alzheimer's on others, but it is possible to be sensitive to one another in the process and partner together to create a meaningful quality of life. A husband reflects on how his priorities in life have shifted for the better: "This can be a time of discovery and growth for both partners. I find in myself a changing sense of what is important in life."

Care Partners Need Their Own Support

Care partners often need to share their feelings with others who understand their unique concerns. Just as you might feel alone sometimes in your experiences with Alzheimer's, your loved ones are at risk of becoming isolated, too. One husband encourages other care partners to seek peer support:

> "You are not alone! You are right in assuming that no one can experience exactly what you do, but there are innumerable people with similar experiences. Finding some of them—some of us—is probably the most important thing you can do in halting the tailspin of your feelings. How? Your local Alzheimer's Association can advise you on this."

Many care partners discuss the need to find education and support services directed toward them so they don't become overwhelmed with too much information. A wife cautions that finding a support group could be counterproductive unless you find one suited to your current concerns:

> "I advise finding a group that is geared toward the earlier stages. It can be depressing to constantly hear of the problems of the later stages of the disease when you are far from there…One should be well-informed of the progression of Alzheimer's, but it serves no useful purpose to dwell on the end stages. It is far better to enjoy the present."

Some people are more private or do not warm up to the idea of attending a support group. There is no one recipe for support. Your care partner needs to determine the kinds of encouragement, resources, strategies, and sources of strength he or she needs to manage effectively and make the most of each day.

Care Partners Need Time Out

Your loved ones may bear the brunt of your feelings as well as their own, and need time out for their own personal or professional interests. Ron Bachrach, who has Alzheimer's, writes:

> "My wife has all of my aggravations and all of her aggravations. I know she cares and that she's with me…but she's suffering, too. And I'm suffering for her because I would like to do more and relieve her of working so hard. She has her own business. Her work is also her therapy to get my problems out of her mind. I'm sure there is some of that."[3]

Although Ron feels helpless to assist his wife, just by acknowledging her stress and respecting her continued work interests, he gives her invaluable support. One wife finds it difficult to get the personal time that she needs: "My husband makes me feel guilty that I want to do something—then I usually end up not doing whatever it is he is complaining about. I find I cannot express my position clearly because it ends in a huge argument. So that causes me stress…"

Take care of your care partners by respecting their need for time out. Bea is concerned about her husband becoming too isolated:

> "Poor Joe, he's stuck with me all of the time. I try to get him to go down in the afternoon and play pool and get away for a few hours because otherwise he's with me constantly…I depend on Joe for everything. I'm isolating him as well as myself, and I'm not being fair to him."[4]

A man with Alzheimer's says, "I urge my wife to get away. My kids are around, so they can help me out if she's gone." He notes that his wife seems more rested and patient when she can get a break for a little while.

Sometimes Your Care Partner's Needs Must Come First

Care partners need time for self care that is both relaxing and restoring. Some may be reluctant to express their own needs, or they feel selfish for taking care of themselves. You and your loved ones must keep in mind that if care partners don't take care of themselves, they are not going to be able to help anyone else. Think of what flight attendants tell passengers on an airplane: If pressure is lost, you must put on your own oxygen mask first before you try to help anyone else. Your loved ones need to find the tools and techniques that allow them to keep breathing deeply and steadily. Self care can be achieved though exercise, quiet time for hobbies, spiritual practices, journaling, meeting friends for coffee, reading a good novel, or any combination of ingredients. In her moving photographic tribute to her husband entitled *I Still Do*, Judith Fox writes:

> "Everyone tells me to take care of myself. Everyone tells me I need to take more time for myself. Everyone tells me that if I

don't take care of myself, I won't be able to properly care for Ed. I know everyone means well. But I need help, not advice. These are some of the things that help me cope: friends, family, and a support group. My personal favorite, though, is mint chocolate chip ice cream."[5]

Ultimately, when your loved ones find greater balance in their own lives, you will likely feel the benefits, too. "Each of us needs time for self, for friends, for fun, for recreation," writes Juanita Tucker. "Fulfilling these needs will not take away from our loved ones. Indeed, it will nourish and enrich us, and enable us to give more."[6]

How You Can Help

With the onset of your memory problems and other symptoms, your care partner will have assumed more responsibilities around the home and in managing other responsibilities. You may wonder what you can do in return. Consider the following:

Offer to Assist with Routine Chores

It may take you longer to do something, but it is important that you offer your help and participate in daily tasks when possible. One man tells his friends in his support group, "I'm teaching myself to take the load off of my wife. I come in now and offer to dry the dishes." When asked how her husband with Alzheimer's shows caring for her, one care partner responded with a big smile, "He brings me my coffee in the morning."

Identify Ways to Work Together

One wife expresses the importance of maintaining open communication: "We talk about our needs each day…We have both accepted the diagnosis, and talking about it is helpful. When problems arise, we try work out a solution together."

Take Steps to Ease Their Stress

You may want to hide your memory problems or stay as independent as possible for fear of becoming a burden. However, this is rarely helpful. If you are having difficulty with an activity that could involve risk to yourself or others, such as managing finances or doing home repairs, accept that others have realistic concerns. Caring for your care partner may mean making sacrifices. Perhaps you let your care partner do the driving, or maybe you give that early-stage program in your community a try even if you'd rather avoid it. Just as the people who care for you are making adjustments and sacrifices, sometimes you will need to, as well. By trying to ease their concerns, you respect their feelings. One man with Alzheimer's advises another: "Be sure you're doing things in a way that doesn't worry your caregiver. It makes me feel better when she's not worried."

Express Your Gratitude and Love

Sometimes the smallest acts are the most helpful. A simple and sincere "thank you" or a warm, appreciative hug expresses your gratitude and care. One daughter says about her mother, "She gives me laughter and 'thank yous' that brighten my day." Never underestimate these very meaningful act of caring. Although memory loss and other symptoms may result in others providing more assistance to you, there are many ways you can give back in return.

In Honor of Those Who Care

You may already extend your gratitude to your care partner. However, some people with Alzheimer's have limited awareness of their symptoms, so loved ones may receive little thanks for their significant efforts to keep life running smoothly. It becomes essential that these caregivers hear praise and appreciation from others who may be more aware of their efforts.

One Thanksgiving, members of the early-stage support group at the Shiley-Marcos Alzheimer's Disease Research Center in San Diego decided to express their gratitude to the loved ones who help them through each day and who make their worlds a better place. Each participant contributed a line in the following poem that was given to their care partners.

My World is a Better Place...
because you're always there by my side when I need you.
because we've shared special memories together.
because of all the things you do for me: find things when I lose them, drive me where I need to go, cook for me.
because you really know me...what I need and what I like.
because you put up with me when I'm feeling grumpy or crotchety, or when I'm wrong about something.
because you give me a hug and a kiss when I need them.
because it's comfortable to be together, even without talking.
because of your unselfishness and the sacrifices you make for me.
My world is a better place because of you.[7]

Take some time to consider how your world is a better place because of others who care. If you do not have an identified care partner, think of a friend or other concerned person who may be trying to better your life at this time. By extending your gratitude and appreciation for those who are caring for you, you become a caregiver in return.

Questions for Discussion

- How do you show respect or concern for your loved ones' feelings? Are you ever insensitive to their feelings?
- How do you respond to your care partner's needs for personal time?
- In what ways are you trying to be helpful to the people who are helping you?

Suggestions for Taking Care of Your Care Partner

- Try to sit down with your care partners or loved ones and discuss the ways that you can be of help or support to them as you work to manage changes and challenges together.

- Make a list of some of the ways you can help your care partners.
- Ask your care partners to make a list of the things they can do for themselves to maintain their well-being. Try to understand when they need to take time out for these self-care activities.
- Write down everything that you appreciate about your care partners, and share your thoughts with them.

Chapter Twenty-Four

Finding and Using Available Community Resources

This chapter provides an overview of organizations, services, and programs that may be helpful to you now in the early stages of Alzheimer's. You cannot always predict what you will need further down the road, and the pathways toward new treatments, services, and care are changing and improving all the time. However, it can be helpful to have a basic understanding of resources that you can access and make use of as needed.

> *Making use of available community services helps you to navigate unfamiliar ground and move forward more smoothly.*

It is Alright to Set Your Own Pace

Everyone seeks and uses resources differently, and there is no one recipe that you and your loved ones have to follow. Well-meaning professionals, family members, and friends have their own ideas about what may be helpful, what steps you need to take, or what they think you need in order to cope effectively. But, each person charts his or her own course through the Alzheimer's experience. Some people want a clear roadmap with planned destinations, good directions, and measurable milestone markers; others prefer to travel day by day, see where the road takes them, and seek assistance when they hit a roadblock and need help to get back on track. You and your loved ones will set your own pace, and it is normal to have times when you are out of step or marching to different drummers. What you do *not* want to do, however, is wait until you are completely out of stamina or are terribly lost in foreign terrain before you signal for help. Most people find that use of available community services helps them to navigate unfamiliar ground and move forward more smoothly.

Helpful Community Resources

The primary programs and services that you and your family can benefit from during the early stages of Alzheimer's include:

- Education programs focused on early-stage symptoms and concerns.
- Early-stage support groups (see Chapter 15).
- Physically and mentally stimulating activities and classes such as adult education lectures or courses, senior fitness programs, or specialized programs designed for people with early-stage Alzheimer's.
- Federally funded university-based Alzheimer's Disease Centers that may have promising research studies, clinical trials, and other programs or services.
- Transportation services, especially if you are no longer driving.
- Legal and financial planning assistance (see Chapter 26).
- Care management services for individuals who live alone or for couples or families needing assistance with accessing and coordinating services, activities, or care (see Chapter 13).

Early-stage educational programs teach attendees the basics of Alzheimer's, and also discuss actions to take now or plans you should make for the future. They usually provide an orientation to services available in the community and are most often sponsored by various Alzheimer's organizations.

Specialized support groups for people with early-stage Alzheimer's and their families are usually six to eight weeks long and have a strong educational component so participants can have a forum to learn and discuss key topics together. Some early-stage support groups are ongoing or have follow-up meetings so families can stay connected.

A small but growing number of communities are also developing innovative programs to engage the interests of people with mild symptoms who want to stay mentally and physically active. Some of these programs include structured cognitive (thinking) stimulation through discussion or mentally challenging games, cultural or recreational outings in the community, volunteer work, or programs for couples to do together. The availability of these programs varies considerably across the country, but as more people become diagnosed with early-stage Alzheimer's or a related disorder, there is a growing need for such programs.

Alzheimer's Disease Centers often provide much more than research. The National Institutes on Aging funds 29 Alzheimer's Disease Centers across the country. These centers enroll people with Alzheimer's and related disorders in research efforts aimed to better understand, prevent, and treat dementias, and they usually provide a multidisciplinary team of physicians, nurses, social workers, and neuropsychologists who can provide invaluable support to research participants and the community. These centers may also be sites for other innovative programs, information, and services for early-stage families.

Where to Find Community Resources

Each community has its own resources, and the easiest way to find them is usually through national organizations that can link you to your regional services. The following organizations can help you find local community resources.

- **The Alzheimer's Association** (800-272-3900 or www.alz.org) is head-quartered in Chicago, Illinois, and maintains regional chapters across the country. Its mission is "to eliminate Alzheimer's disease through the advancement of research; to provide and enhance care and support for all affected; and to reduce the risk of dementia through the promotion of brain health." Nationwide chapters provide core services to families in their communities, including support groups, consultation with social workers or other professionals, information and referral services, and educational programs. Each chapter is responsible for a geographic region that can be as specific as a single city or span the breadth of two states. By calling the national number you may be routed directly to your local chapter.
- **Eldercare Locater** (800-677-1116 or www.eldercare.gov) is a nationwide program that can connect you with a broad range of services that may be available in your community. Although these services are not specific to Alzheimer's, they are widely used by families as needed. You may find assistance with locating senior centers; adult day services; care management; legal and financial help; home care services; and a variety of community programs that could be helpful.
- **Alzheimer's Disease Education and Referral (ADEAR)** (800-438-4380 or www.nia.nih.gov/Alzheimers) staff can inform you of any federally funded Alzheimer's Disease Centers in your region. If your region of the country is not near one of the 29 centers, ADEAR can still provide a great deal of written and online information about Alzheimer's that can be very helpful to families.
- **Family Caregiver Alliance** (800-445-8106 or www.caregiver.org) is a nationwide organization devoted to caregivers and can be a valuable source of information for your loved ones. The Alliance provides information through its family care navigator on a wide range of services available in your community. It also has helpful materials for caregiver education and support, as well as innovative online support services.
- **The Alzheimer's Foundation of America (AFA)** (866-232-8484 or

www.alzfdn.org) is a national organization, headquartered in New York City, that partners with more than 1,200 organizations nationwide "to provide optimal care and services to individuals confronting dementia, and to their caregivers and families—through member organizations dedicated to improving quality of life." You can contact AFA or view its Web site for helpful information and to learn about any partnering organizations in your community.

If You Live in a Rural Area

Citizens in rural areas can face unique challenges in obtaining services. There may be limited access to specialists and few transportation services to assist with traveling the distance required to receive assistance. The organizations listed above can all be helpful in informing rural families of available services. Some Alzheimer's Association chapters have special rural outreach programs, as do some regional universities, Alzheimer's Disease Centers, or Public Health Departments that may have specific grants or other funds to serve rural populations.

If you live in a rural community, you may not have as many specialized Alzheimer's services easily available to you, but you may find valuable assistance through other senior services agencies, religious organizations, care management, or home healthcare agencies that serve your area. While some people maintain a close-knit sense of community in rural areas and rely on one another for all different kinds of assistance and neighbor-to-neighbor support, others may find that there is a strong sense of independence and autonomy in residents of rural regions, and it may be harder to acknowledge any need for outside information or assistance.

If you are informed about Alzheimer's symptoms and make use of available services you may actually increase your independence and better manage your circumstances. It is not a weakness to ask for information or help; in fact, it usually conveys sound judgment and resourceful problem-solving skills.

Questions for Discussion

- Have you or your loved ones contacted any of the organizations listed in this chapter? If so, did you get the information or assistance you were seeking?
- Do you think you could benefit from any of the types of programs or services listed in this chapter? If so, what would be helpful to you at this time?
- Are you reluctant to seek information or services pertaining to Alzheimer's? If so, why?
- Have you ever made use of community services or resources at any other time in your life? If so, what was your experience?

Suggestions for Making the Best Use of Community Resources

- Learn what is available so you can be informed about potentially helpful resources for you and your loved ones. Share what you learn with each other, but also respect any differing needs for information and services.
- Contact the organizations listed in this chapter for information. Create a file so you have resources at hand if needed.
- Pace yourself. It is not necessary to read everything or make use of all resources now. You can refer back to your file as needed when concerns arise.
- If your national or community organizations do not have the information or services you need, tell them what is missing. Many educational materials, programs, and services are developed because someone speaks up, makes the need known, and asks for help.

Chapter Twenty-Five

Creating and Communicating with Your Healthcare Team

Everyone has varied experiences with healthcare systems throughout the course of their lives. Some have had positive experiences over the years in obtaining preventative health screenings or the care needed with the onset of a medical problem. Others have had a harder time getting necessary care or have had unfavorable experiences with care providers. Some people have had little reason over their lifetime to see a physician and have enjoyed exceptionally good health, while others are more familiar with accessing medical care needed for a variety of concerns.

> *"You would be wise to take a supportive companion with you to important appointments."*

Getting to Know Your Team Players

With the onset of Alzheimer's or a related disorder, it is essential to form a healthcare team who can help you manage symptoms and overall health, and work with you to maintain a good quality of life. This team can partner with you to evaluate problems and address concerns as they arise. Effective communication between you, your loved ones, and these team players is an essential component to living your best with Alzheimer's.

The treatment and care of Alzheimer's symptoms can involve professionals from a variety of healthcare disciplines who each has expertise in a different area. The following are the most common members of an Alzheimer's care team.

Physicians

Physicians form the core of your medical team, and the evaluation and treatment of Alzheimer's can include different types of specialists. Many people discuss their initial concerns with memory loss or other symptoms with their primary care doctor or geriatrician. If this person is well known to you and understands your medical history, you can more readily discuss any memory changes or other problems you are having now. If this doctor is new to you, he or she will need to have a full understanding of your medical history and how it may be impacting your current circumstances.

Your primary care doctor might do the complete evaluation and treatment of your symptoms, or you could be referred to a neurologist, a specialist in the brain and nervous system. A neurologist should be well versed in the latest means of diagnosing and treating Alzheimer's symptoms and can work with your primary care doctor to ensure that you have a thorough evaluation and are receiving appropriate medications for treating your symptoms. You may only see a neurologist once or twice as part of your initial evaluation or, depending on your insurance, you may decide to use a neurologist as your primary doctor for Alzheimer's-related problems.

Psychiatrists specifically treat mood and behavioral disturbances, and they can play a helpful role in your medical team as needed. Some psychiatrists specialize in geriatrics, including the treatment of Alzheimer's and related disorders. A psychiatrist can be consulted if you or your loved ones are concerned about significant changes in your mood, such as depression, irritability, or ongoing suspiciousness. Psychiatrists can also be helpful in evaluating disruptive changes in your behavior, such as sleep disturbance. It is essential that any psychiatrist on your team have expertise in Alzheimer's, however, as some commonly prescribed medications for mood and behavioral disturbances can have other risks or side effects when given to people with Alzheimer's and related disorders.

Nurses and Physician Assistants

Nurses have college- or graduate-level academic degrees and may have additional certificates or licenses that represent specialties or authorizations for providing types of medical care. A nurse can be an important liaison between you and your physician by helping to coordinate your care, communicate information, and provide the additional teaching or instructions necessary for you to understand your condition and follow the doctor's treatment plan. Nurse practitioners have additional graduate-level training and licensing do more comprehensive patient care or, in some cases, prescribe medications under a physician's supervision. Physician's assistants work in a similar capacity as nurse practitioners. Most have a graduate degree and provide some amount of medical care under a physician's supervision. Physician's assistants are most often employed in hospitals and medical clinics.

Neuropsychologists

Neuropsychologists obtain a doctorate in psychology (a PhD) and specialize in understanding the brain and its role in cognition (thinking) and behavior. Neuropsychologists perform their evaluations through a series of paper-and-pencil tests as well as other measures that test your thinking, including your memory, judgment, problem solving, and language abilities. You may be referred to a neuropsychologist as part of a comprehensive medical evaluation to help determine the specific cause of your memory loss or other cognitive symptoms. A neuropsychologist (or your neurologist or geriatrician) can help you and your family understand how affected regions of your brain can result in some of the symptoms you are experiencing. This can help everyone take symptoms less personally.

Social Workers

Social workers have college- or graduate-level academic degrees in the profession of social work and may also have additional training and licensing that allows them to do private counseling or therapy. Some social workers specialize in geriatrics or Alzheimer's services and can be very helpful in working with you and your loved ones to obtain community resources, develop positive strategies and coping skills for daily living, and manage the emotional and logistical challenges of living with symptoms. Social workers may be able to meet with or you or your care partner individually, together, or as a family. You can find social workers through community Alzheimer's organizations or your medical care practice and can ask to be referred for a consultation so you can become familiar with the social worker's role on your team.

It may take some time to put your professional team together, but it is important to have a few key reliable, respectful, and caring professionals to seek assistance or counsel from as needed. Lynn's husband was diagnosed with Alzheimer's in his mid 50s. She says, "One the most positive things we have encountered is the caring, compassion, and willingness to do more than expected from all of the professionals—from doctor to social worker—that are specifically in this field."

Preparing for an Appointment

Many people feel rushed in their appointments with healthcare providers, but if you come well-organized and prepared for your appointment, you can make better use of the limited time.

- Schedule your appointments during the time of day when you are at your best. Try to be well rested before your appointment.
- Make a list of your questions or problems that you want to discuss with your healthcare provider. Be specific about any symptoms or concerns, and provide examples when possible. Your care partner may have different perspectives or observations about your symptoms to share during the appointment.

- Bring a list of all medications you are taking, including vitamins or supplements, or bring them with you. This ensures that your doctor is up to date on your medications and can monitor any side effects.

Why You Don't Want to Go to Appointments Alone

Some people are accustomed to going to their medical appointments alone or may value their privacy concerning their health care. Others appreciate the support or practical assistance of a loved one during medical appointments and are comfortable including others in their appointments. With the onset of memory loss of other Alzheimer's symptoms, it is important to take someone with you to your medical appointments. Memory problems can interfere with your ability to accurately describe your problems to a doctor. One man tells friends in his support group: "I try to appreciate that my caregiver often has to be my interpreter. A good caregiver can be an important communicator to tell others what is going on. They are good observers. A lot of us don't tell the doctor everything. We forget what we forget."

Memory loss can also make it difficult to remember the details of any explanations or instructions your doctor provides to you during the appointment. Philip Aldertions recounts:

> "When I went to see the specialist, my wife came along to keep me company. After we had seen him, she remembered in detail many of the things that I had forgotten. I was so pleased that she had accompanied me. She is now invited to all of my appointments. You, too, would be wise to take a supportive companion with you to important appointments."[1]

Developing Effective Communication with Your Doctor

Good communication between you and your doctor forms the foundation for your care. While some may rely on the doctor to determine the problem and find the solution, your doctor can be of limited assistance without you and your loved ones first communicating your concerns. Frequently, your doctor may ask your care partner to help describe problems. This may result in you feeling angry or left out of the conversation. Joan Cahill, a retired nurse who has Alzheimer's, says, "There are times when I have gone to my doctor's office and been ignored. The doctors sometimes have to be reminded to talk with me, not just my family."[2]

Sometimes your loved ones might want to talk alone with the doctor about their own concerns with your symptoms. This is especially true if you tend to become defensive or distressed with discussion of these problems. They may also have their own personal stressors they would rather discuss with the doctor privately. In general, however, it is most productive if everyone can meet together and discuss matters in a way that respects each person's perspective. If your loved ones have their own concerns, they may need to communicate them to the doctor's nurse or the doctor via a private phone call, letter, or fax prior to the meeting rather than leaving you out of important discussions during the appointment.

You are the patient, and you may need to take some responsibility for making your voice heard. Gloria Sterin reflects on a visit with her neurologist:

> "My husband was with me, and when the doctor came to see me, and before I had anything to say to him, the two of them were having a virtual medical meeting on Alzheimer's, while I listened, getting more and more frustrated because I was forgetting what I wanted to ask and they both seemed to have forgotten that I was there. I felt as though I was being treated like a child, expected to sit quietly while the adults had their important discussion, which I could not be expected to understand. At a later session I got my act together, and when they started their conversation, I barged in and told the neurologist I had questions. He pushed back his chair, listened carefully, and answered very fully. In retrospect, it may or may not be true that he made some erroneous assumptions, but my failure to speak out sooner was just as much, if not more, to blame."[3]

Your healthcare team is there to partner with you to address any concerns that may arise. If you do not have effective communication with any member of your team, you have a right to find a replacement. If you feel rushed or are uncomfortable talking with your physician about certain symptoms or private matters, try to share your concerns with a nurse, physician's assistant, or a social worker who will take responsibility for conveying your concerns to the physician. Keep in mind that strict confidentiality laws often prohibit team members from speaking with one another without your or your loved one's permission.

Questions for Discussion

- What has been your experience with the types of healthcare professionals listed in this chapter? How has each one been helpful or unhelpful to you?
- Are you able to communicate effectively with your healthcare team? If not, what are the challenges?
- How do you feel about having a loved one with you during your appointments? Is it helpful? Is it ever hurtful?

Suggestions for Making the Most of Your Healthcare Team

- Make a list of your healthcare team players and keep it in one central location for easy access.
- Make sure you have good communication with at least one physician, nurse, and social worker so you can make use of these team members as needed.
- Sometimes others are more aware of changes in your mood or behavior than you are. Try to trust loved ones when they suggest you seek medical attention or counsel.
- Don't hesitate to ask clarifying questions if the healthcare provider's explanations or instructions are unclear. Write down all information or

ask for special written instructions from a nurse or physician's assistant.

- Make sure your doctor has a copy of your Healthcare Proxy document (see chapter 26).
- Obtain a copy of the free booklet *Partnering With Your Doctor: A Guide for Persons with Memory Problems and Their Care Partners* from the Alzheimer's Association by calling 800-292-3900.

Chapter Twenty-Six

Helpful Legal, Financial and Long-Term Planning

Everyone can benefit from some amount of advanced legal and financial planning, and the recommendations discussed in this chapter are certainly not limited to Alzheimer's. No one knows when a sudden accident or event might occur that could make it difficult to express your needs or wishes. Being proactive gives you the opportunity to make informed decisions affecting your future.

> *"I want to be part of shaping my future.....I want to be able to express my wishes for as long as I can."*

Sooner Is Better Than Later

With the onset of Alzheimer's symptoms, it is important to communicate about your values and preferences concerning legal and financial planning early on so that your wishes are honored to the extent possible. Symptoms may eventually have an impact on the abilities necessary for sound planning and decision-making. For example, memory loss can result in forgetting to deposit checks or pay monthly bills. Challenges with organizing and processing information or with problem solving can result in difficulty managing a checkbook, tracking investments, or making legal or financial transactions. For some people, affected judgment may result in mismanagement of finances, irrational spending, or being taken advantage of by disreputable individuals or organizations. While these issues may not currently seem urgent to you, it is wise to make decisions now before your symptoms advance and affect your ability to make logical, informed decisions that are consistent with your values and preferences.

Effective Teamwork and Communication

Respectful and open communication is essential when discussing decisions about legal and financial planning. "There has to be a lot of trust," says Betty, who is newly diagnosed with Alzheimer's. "By having enough trust, you can bear a lot of things and make decisions that are really mutual."[1]

If you have a positive history of trust and communication with a care partner, you can build on this as you address these new decisions in life. If you have been accustomed to being independent, in control, and making decisions on your own, you may be challenged by this new need to involve others in decisions that are personal and significant. This is all the more reason to take action now so you can make your wishes known and be in charge of how your affairs are managed. "I want to be part of shaping my own future," says Frank. "Between my wife and my family, we try to stay open and honest and realistic. I want to be able to express my wishes for as long as I can."[2]

The Basics of Legal Planning

Most legal planning involves the creation of a will and/or a trust, appointment of durable powers of attorney, and consideration of any future need for a conservator or legal guardian. The following are the basic components of legal planning.

Living Trust

In a living trust, you outline how your property and financial assets are to be managed during your life as well as at the time of your death. A living trust is often advisable for individuals or couples who have property or assets that require more detailed management, or when you have specific preferences for how assets are managed or spent while you are alive. Living trusts require an attorney to help you organize all of the necessary information and to write up the document according to legal standards.

Last Will and Testament

This document outlines how you want your assets or personal belongings distributed to individuals or organizations at the time of your death and may be included in a living trust. A will includes your appointment of an executor to be in charge of carrying out your preferences as outlined. Forms for a last will and testament can be found in stationary stores or online, but if you put together a will on your own, it is advisable to have an attorney examine it to make sure it is completed appropriately and is legally valid.

Durable Power of Attorney

Durable power of attorney can be included in a living trust or may be a separate document. In this document, you appoint one or more individuals (a deeply trusted family member, friend, or professional) as your agent to manage your finances and make decisions about your property during your life if you are no longer capable. Your agent could eventually have authority to write checks from your accounts, manage your investments, sell your property, or make other significant choices concerning your estate. *Durable* power of attorney is preferable to a regular power of attorney because it remains in effect if you are not able to make these decisions on your own.

Durable power of attorney is a serious document that affords someone else considerable control over your financial affairs at a point when you may be most vulnerable. Think carefully about whom you appoint to this trusted position. Appoint someone who is reliable and sound in their decision making and who will be respectful and caring concerning your needs and wishes. Without such a document, you are at greater risk of being taken advantage of by others who may not have your best financial interests in mind.

Durable power of attorney forms may be available in stationary stores or online, but due to the significance of this document, an attorney should draw up or review the document to ensure that your rights and welfare are adequately protected.

Healthcare Proxy (or Durable Power of Attorney for Healthcare)

This document allows you to appoint a person as your agent, as well as one or more alternates, to make healthcare decisions for you if you are unable to make them for yourself. Many hospitals, and indeed some states, require that any adult patient have a healthcare proxy document on file in order for families to participate in healthcare decision making or obtain medical information about their loved one. This document outlines your wishes concerning use or withholding of life support, organ donation, and other details concerning your healthcare preferences. In the event that you have a sudden accident or are not able to communicate your own wishes, your agent has authority to choose medical providers, make long-term care decisions, and carry out your healthcare wishes.

Healthcare Proxy forms are often available through your local hospital or healthcare provider's office. You may also be able to download your state's specific form online. These forms are fairly straightforward and generally do not require the assistance of an attorney to complete. It is important that your appointed agents and your healthcare providers have a copy of your Healthcare Proxy.

Guardians and Conservators

If you have not completed powers of attorney and made arrangements for others to manage your affairs if needed, you may lose important decision-making authority. If your symptoms advance or you are not able to make decisions on your own behalf, a court may step in and appoint a guardian or conservator to manage your affairs. Although the appointed person might be a family member or close acquaintance, in some cases an outside agency or professional is appointed. Completing your powers of attorney avoids this more complex and often costly route.

Finding an Attorney and Preparing for a Meeting

An attorney specializing in "elder law" is usually the most informed choice for families facing Alzheimer's. Elder law attorneys are qualified to discuss estate planning, including powers of attorney, trusts, wills, and the details of qualifying for any financial or long-term care benefits. An elder law attorney can also help you discuss options for a personal advocate if you do not have a care partner and are at some point unable to direct your own care needs. Your local senior center, Area Agency on Aging, or Alzheimer's organization should have referrals for reputable elder law attorneys. You can also locate an attorney through National Academy of Elder Law Attorneys, Inc., at www.naela.org.

Before you meet with an attorney, ask about the documents you should bring with you to the appointment. You may need personal identification records, a marriage certificate, records of any property and assets, insurance policies, or other information related to the specific purpose of your consultation. List any questions you have in advance so you can address them during your meeting. You will make the best use of your visit if you arrive organized and well prepared.

If You Cannot Afford an Attorney

If you cannot afford to consult an attorney, assistance may be available through a legal aid society in your community. Some attorneys work on a sliding scale basis or pro bono (free of charge) for exceptional circumstances, and your state bar association may have referrals to appropriate attorneys. If you do not have considerable assets or a complex estate, you and your care partner may be able to draw up a common will on your own. Some senior centers provide classes or workshops on legal and financial planning, including appropriate forms. You can complete as much as possible on your own and then have a brief meeting with an attorney to make sure your documents are in order.

To learn about any free legal aid programs available in your community see Law Help at www.lawhelp.org.

The Essentials of Financial Planning

Many people worry about the expenses of living with Alzheimer's. Some people have to retire early due to the onset of symptoms, while others may be concerned about how to plan for future care needs. Financial planning is unique to each person's circumstances, but there are some general components to keep in mind.

Social Security and Disability Benefits

If you are no longer employed, you may derive some income from Social Security or disability benefits. Social Security is a federal government benefit that is generally collected after age 65. Since many people with Alzheimer's are diagnosed later in life, most are already receiving Social Security income. The monthly amount will depend on the years that you (or your spouse) worked and the amount that was paid into Social Security during employment.

If you had to retire prior to age 65 due to the onset of symptoms, you may be eligible for disability benefits through your employer, your state disability program, or through the federal Social Security Disability system. File for any disability benefits as soon as you are no longer working, as there are time limits for some disability programs. It can also take considerable time between the date you file for disability and the time you begin to receive your benefits, so it is wise to act sooner rather than later to secure any available resources.

If your income is low or you did not pay into the Social Security system, you may be eligible for monthly Supplemental Security Income (SSI) through the federal government based on your Alzheimer's diagnosis. Contact your local Alzheimer's organization or senior center for referrals to social workers, advocates, or other specialists who can help you as needed with this potentially confusing process.

For more information about Social Security benefits, contact Social Security Administration at 800-772-1213 or www. ssa.gov.

Planning for Long-Term Care Expenses

Long-term care expenses refer to costs associated with services while you are living at home or the payment for care provided in an assisted-living or long-term care home. Long-term care expenses are paid for either privately (with your own funds), through insurance policies, or through the federal Medicaid benefit. Most health insurance policies, including Medicare, do not pay for the long-term care expenses usually associated with Alzheimer's, but check with your company to determine any benefits that may be available to you.

If you bought a separate long-term care insurance policy prior to the onset of Alzheimer's, it likely covers some of the expenses of in-home or out-of-home care, and check with your insurance agent to review when this policy may be of help. Long-term care insurance policies are very hard to obtain once a diagnosis has been made, however. Likewise, if you have a life insurance policy, it might help with expenses during your life, and your insurance agent can advise you of specifics.

If you are married, federal guidelines have been established to keep your spouse from becoming impoverished by the long-term care costs associated with Alzheimer's. Couples must generally pay for long-term care costs out of pocket until they spend down to a certain income and asset level. Once they have paid their share of expenses, the federal government supplements long-term care costs through the Medicaid program. Each state has set its own guidelines for this program.

If you are not married, you need to use your own assets to pay for your long-term care costs. Once your assets are exhausted, or if you do not have savings or resources, Medicaid covers most long-term care needs. Each state is unique in the kinds of services available to low-income disabled individuals. Both married couples and single individuals should consult with their regional Alzheimer's organizations for referrals to elder-law attorneys or social service agencies that can clarify eligibility for medical benefits.

Veteran's Benefits

If you are a veteran, it is important to check with your local Veteran's Administration hospital or Department of Veteran's Affairs to determine whether any veteran's benefits will help with long-term care expenses. Coverage may depend on the specifics of your service, but if you are eligible for benefits, they can be helpful with expenses related to your Alzheimer's care both in and out of the home.

Making Decisions about Future Care Needs

People can live with mild symptoms of Alzheimer's for many years, and it is difficult to predict how symptoms will advance. However, it is important that you have the opportunity to make your wishes known about a wide range of decisions affecting your care and well-being in the event your symptoms worsen.

In a study called, *Making Hard Choices: Respecting Both Voices* conducted at the Family Caregiver Alliance in San Francisco, California, researchers found that people with early- to moderate-stage Alzheimer's or a related disorder were reliably able to express their values and wishes in six key areas, including healthcare, finances, personal care, social activities, living arrangements, and the possibility of living in a nursing home. They were also able to appropriately choose a person to make decisions for them in these areas when necessary. It is important to note that researchers in this study also found that care partners were not always aware of some of the values and care preferences expressed by their loved one.[3] Try to have discussions about any future care concerns and wishes now, and write down your care preferences.

Legal, financial, and long-term planning is an important step in being proactive about managing Alzheimer's. These issues are often complex, dependent on personal circumstance, and vary somewhat, depending on where you live. Seek professional assistance to make sure you understand all of the steps in this planning process as well as any available benefits so you can move forward knowing you have planned the best you can.

Questions for Discussion

- Is there a history of positive teamwork and communication between you and your loved ones concerning financial and healthcare decision-making? What helps or hinders your communication or ability to work together?
- Have you completed appropriate legal planning, including powers of attorney? If not, what are your concerns about completing these documents?
- Do you have concerns about potential expenses associated with Alzheimer's care? If so, have you been able to talk to someone about these issues?

Suggestions for Taking the Next Steps in Planning

- Identify your primary and alternate care partners, and make sure they are comfortable respecting your financial planning and healthcare wishes. Discuss any concerns you have now so you can assure you are working effectively as a team.
- Review with your care partner any impact of Alzheimer's on your ability to manage your own financial affairs. Discuss at what point it might be helpful to have your designated power of attorney step in to assist as needed. If you are in disagreement about the timing or need for help, get an outside opinion from your doctor or other Alzheimer's specialist.
- If you have any concerns about how others are managing your finances or making decisions about your care, or if you feel that you are being taken advantage of in any way, talk with a doctor, social worker, or your local Alzheimer's organization to make sure someone is addressing your concern.

Chapter Twenty-Seven

Maintaining an Ongoing Quality of Life

Many people with early-stage Alzheimer's, and their loved ones, have concerns about how to continue having a meaningful and satisfying life in the face of an incurable medical condition. Some people report that the diagnosis left them feeling as if life was suddenly over, with little hope for a future. You will experience many changes in your life as a result of Alzheimer's, but your life is far from over. Quality of life refers to your ability to continue to experience satisfaction and well-being. What constitutes good quality of life varies from person to person, but is usually influenced by the people, activities, or experiences that give you the most pleasure, as well as your overall physical and emotional health.

> *Identify the actions, activities, and attitudes that give you and your loved ones satisfaction and meaning.*

The Ingredients of Good Quality of Life

You and your loved ones ultimately determine the ingredients that contribute to your ongoing quality of life, but there are some important general considerations. The research of Rebecca Logsdon, PhD, at the University of Washington in Seattle suggests that individuals with Alzheimer's report a better quality of life when they do the following:

- Focus on their abilities versus their losses.
- Have positive relationships with others versus dissatisfying ones.
- Maintain some of their previously enjoyed activities versus giving up on them entirely.[1]

These core principles can provide an important foundation for maintaining quality of life for both you and your care partner and provide wise counsel for all involved in the Alzheimer's experience.

Participants of an early-stage Alzheimer's support group facilitated by Darby Morhardt, LCSW at Northwestern University's Alzheimer's Disease Center in Chicago, Illinois, support these findings with their own specific reflections. Below, they offer ten ideas for enhancing quality of life.[2] Others with Alzheimer's also voice their opinions throughout this chapter. As you read these messages from your peers, think about which ideas you agree with and how you may be experiencing these suggestions in your own life. These concepts apply equally well to care partners who are trying to maintain their own well-being.

Remain Active and Involved

Meaningful activity contributes significantly to quality of life and often generates positive feelings of purpose, engagement, and belonging. Many people with Alzheimer's continue to enjoy a number of activities that can take their minds off symptoms. "I find that keeping busy is very important," says Jenny. "You have to keep moving forward."[3] Social isolation can reduce quality of life, so try to have some of your activity include others. It is important that you be able to make choices about the types of activities you participate in and that you open your mind to new possibilities (see Chapter 17).

What do you do to feel active and involved in life?

Make Sure You Have Support

Support may mean different things to different people, but generally it includes the people or actions that help you more effectively continue on in the face of hardship. Barbara tells professionals in Great Britain about the importance of support: "Support is the key to my leading as normal a life as possible—knowing and treating me as the person I still am, giving me room to live."[4]

You may receive support from affirming family, friends, a caring professional, or a spiritual faith. Some appreciate a peer group with whom they can exchange encouragement or camaraderie with others "in the same boat" (see Chapter 15). Many people with Alzheimer's acknowledge the invaluable support of a care partner who helps them make it through each day. Early-stage Alzheimer's support group members in Ingle Farm, Australia, tell their loved ones, "We acknowledge that there are times when we don't express our appreciation. We do appreciate your help and support very much!"[5]

Who provides support to you when you need it? How do you give support to others?

Take Care of Yourself Physically and Mentally

Personal health is important for both you and your loved ones. You can maintain better quality of life by eating well, getting enough sleep, and staying physically active.

How well do you take care of your health?

Remain Positive

Although this tip may seem easier said than followed, there are always positive aspects of life to acknowledge. Perhaps you had an enjoyable conversation with a friend, saw your grandchild take her first steps, discovered a park you had never visited before, or felt the warm sun after too many days of rain. When speaking as a panelist at a California conference on Alzheimer's, William tells the audience: "When I was growing up, I saw a sign that said 'As you ramble through life, whatever your goal, keep your eye on the doughnut and not on the hole!'"

Find things to be grateful for each day and talk about them with others. You may be surprised at how one positive thing can lead to another and begin to offset the harder times.

What helps you feel positive?

Accept Your Limitations

It is important to realize that you might not be able to do things in exactly the same way that you used to, and being patient with yourself is important to quality of life.

How well do you accept your limitations? What are your strengths?

Maintain a Familiar Environment, Routine and Sense of Organization

Many people discuss strategies for keeping track of things and staying organized. Putting things away in the same place, maintaining a calendar, or staying on a familiar route while walking are all examples of ways people adapt to memory loss and maintain quality of life. Jan talks about her family routines: "We've made my life more of a habit. When we walk, we walk the same path, we eat dinner at the same time, and that helps make things a lot safer."[6]

Are there any familiar routines that help to maintain or improve your quality of life?

Take Safety Precautions

It is helpful to get assistance or be cautious in areas that pose risk, such as cooking or taking long walks alone. You can feel more secure and confident if you take precautions as needed. Letty Tennis was diagnosed in her 50s with Alzheimer's and writes in her diary, "I can't handle medication. I'd never remember from five minutes after having taken something. All drugs are now hidden, and my husband gives me my meds."[7] (See Chapter 11 for a discussion of ways to maximize your safety.)

Have you or your care partner taken any actions or precautions to enhance your safety?

Don't Be Afraid to Try Something New

Establishing routine and paying attention to safety does not mean that you can't explore new experiences. Think of different things to do or places to see. Some people take up a new hobby. One Chicago support group participant has started sketching: "Often people approach me when I'm sketching and ask how I can do that. I've come close to saying, 'Well first, you have to have Alzheimer's!'"[8]

Have you tried anything new lately?

Maintain as Much Control for as Long as Possible

You cannot always control Alzheimer's symptoms, but there are choices that you can make each day that afford you some control. One woman states, "There are little tricks that you learn. Once you get used to the idea that you're not a free agent anymore, there's lots of things you can work out to make life manageable and keep some independence."[9] Making basic daily decisions such as which restaurant to go to or what movie to see helps regain some feelings of influence in life. Others find that planning for the future, including expressing values and preferences for care, is an important part of maintaining control. Brenda Hounam says, "Being proactive allows you to take control of your life, which is a win-win situation—in gaining control you are in a position to not only improve the quality of your life, but also to live a purposeful life."[10]

In what ways do you have control or decision-making choices in your daily life? In what ways might you also need to let go of some control to maintain your or your loved one's quality of life?

Find Ways to Modify Attitudes and Advocate for Public Policy Change

More people are showing the public that it is possible to have Alzheimer's and also have a good quality of life. At a town hall forum sponsored by the Alzheimer's Association, one person says, "If we can communicate, we can educate the public, we can educate our friends, we can educate our families. It's really important that we talk about this…so there isn't this big stigma about Alzheimer's disease."[11] Certainly any attempts to reduce stigma also go a long way in improving the quality of life for people with Alzheimer's. There are many ways to make a difference (see Chapter 18).

Have you said or done anything to advocate on behalf of yourself or others with Alzheimer's?

Staying Young at Heart

You may not agree with all of these tips for maintaining quality of life, or you may have some of your own to add. Many people with Alzheimer's acknowledge the importance of a good sense of humor and the ability to enjoy simple pleasures that lighten their spirit and make them feel young at heart. When asked, "What do you do to stay young at heart?" People with Alzheimer's gave the following diverse answers:

- I walk by the ocean and dig my feet in the wet sand.
- I stay in bed in the morning as long as I want!
- Anything having to do with chocolate keeps me feeling young at heart.
- A good cup of coffee, tea, or Schnapps gives me a boost.
- Being with children keeps me young at heart. I'm drawn to them.
- I search out old items on the computer and re-read about history. It takes me back.
- Music makes my heart sing. I love classical music especially.
- I played football in college. Sometimes it's like being there again when I watch a game on TV.
- I was a high-school swimmer, so doing laps now at the YMCA makes me feel young at heart—except I get out of breath more easily![12]

What helps you feel young at heart?

Maintaining ongoing quality of life in the early stages of Alzheimer's involves making a conscious effort to identify the actions, activities, and attitudes that give you and your loved ones satisfaction and meaning. Alzheimer's can help you to focus and consider what is truly most important to you and your loved ones, and taking time to pause and reflect is a first step in maintaining and improving your quality of life.

Questions for Discussion

- Which of the Chicago support group members' ten ideas for enhancing quality of life do you most agree with? Are there any ideas you don't agree with?
- What improves your quality of life? What improves your loved one's quality of life?
- What detracts from or reduces your quality of life? What detracts from or reduces your loved one's quality of life?

Suggestions for Maintaining and Improving Quality of Life

- Make a list of the activities, people, attitudes, and experiences that contribute to your quality of life and continue to build on them. Suggest that your loved ones do the same.
- Make a list of the activities, people, attitudes, and experiences that reduce your quality of life. Suggest that your loved ones do the same. Try to reduce any negative influences that are within your control.
- Discuss with your loved ones the ways that you can contribute to each other's quality of life, and make those "young at heart" moments more frequent.

Chapter Twenty-Eight

Progress and Trends in Treatment and Care

For every person living with Alzheimer's, there are countless others attempting to discover or deliver methods of providing effective treatment and respectful, compassionate care. There is no cure for Alzheimer's, but there are many different forms of treatment. While most people assume that treatment means medical intervention, treatment can also include the use of effective strategies for living with symptoms and maintaining well-being so that people with Alzheimer's and their care partners experience a meaningful quality of life. Ultimately, the most effective treatment for Alzheimer's combines progress in both science and society in a hopeful and helpful partnership.

> *"A person with Alzheimer's is many more things than just their diagnosis. Each person is a whole human being."*

Currently Approved Medications May Improve Symptoms

Scientists continue to work to find more effective medicines to treat Alzheimer's symptoms. The medications that are currently available cannot stop the progression of your symptoms, but they do aim to provide some improvement in your memory and other thinking abilities for a limited period of time.

Neurotransmitters are the chemicals in the brain that relay messages between nerve cells, and acetylcholine is a neurotransmitter important for memory. Alzheimer's reduces levels of this important chemical. Current Alzheimer's medications, such as Aricept, Exelon, and Razadyne, aim to maintain necessary levels of acetylcholine and improve your thinking and functioning.

Up to half of those who take these medications respond favorably and feel a small, but positive improvement in their memory, language skills, and ability to do routine tasks within a few months of starting on a drug. Others have uncomfortable side effects including nausea, dizziness, or diarrhea and cannot tolerate the drugs, or experience no real benefit from taking them. A fourth approved medication, Namenda, also has a limited but positive effect on memory performance for some people by targeting the brain chemical glutamate, which is associated with learning and memory. Namenda is often prescribed in combination with one of the previously mentioned medications.

Many physicians prescribe one or more of these medications when Alzheimer's is diagnosed, and some people stay on the treatment for a number of years. For many families, it is difficult to discern any dramatic beneficial effect from the treatment, but perhaps symptoms would be worse or progress more rapidly without the medication. Many people also feel encouraged by being proactive and doing whatever is possible to help themselves live more effectively with Alzheimer's. One woman states:

> "There's been a slight improvement or arrest in progress…and that must be accountable to something, maybe because it's being tackled, maybe because of the drugs, maybe it's both…Maybe it's also me facing up to things and making an effort."[1]

The Importance of Managing Other Health Conditions

Treatment of other medical conditions is essential to the treatment of Alzheimer's. Heart disease, vascular disease, diabetes, viruses or infections, depression, and a host of other medical conditions can all worsen Alzheimer's symptoms, sometimes dramatically. Preventing or managing other medical conditions and maintaining overall physical well-being is an essential part of your treatment plan. Most doctors encourage regular exercise, healthy eating habits, socially and mentally stimulating activity, and routine physical checkups in their prescription for living your best with Alzheimer's.

Your care partner should watch for any sudden or dramatic changes in your mood, symptoms, or physical health, and notify your doctor immediately. Don't automatically assume that sudden changes are due to advancing Alzheimer's and that there is nothing to be done. Other health problems should be ruled out and treated if possible. If your Alzheimer's results in a persistent and troubling mood or behavior that is disturbing to you or your care partner and cannot be addressed through any other means, your doctor may be able to prescribe medication to treat the problem.

Education and Support Are a Form of Treatment

Most people with Alzheimer's and their families can have improved quality of life by learning strategies for dealing with challenges through effective communication, modifications to their routines and activities, accessing various kinds of support, engaging in activity that focuses on remaining strengths, and maintaining their physical and emotional health. There are a growing number of programs through regional Alzheimer's organizations aimed at helping you and your loved ones better understand Alzheimer's and develop adaptive lifestyles. Many educational programs are directed specifically to care partners who are trying to learn effective approaches to partnering with you in managing memory loss and other symptoms while also maintaining their own well-being. Never underestimate that your and your loved ones' efforts to access available resources, develop creative strategies, and maintain your sense of humor are some of the most effective treatments available.

Innovative Approaches in Long-Term Care

Many people with early-stage Alzheimer's wonder what the future holds and how they will be cared for if their symptoms advance. Some may fear the indignity of advanced symptoms or have negative memories of a nursing home in which a parent or loved one resided. There is much encouraging progress being made in caring for people throughout the continuum of Alzheimer's. Professional care is becoming more creative, effective, and dignified, and increasingly professional caregivers and long-term-care home staff are being trained in these affirming practices. You can feel more at ease about the future knowing that if you do need to leave your home at some point, you can be cared for by compassionate people in a creative and life-affirming setting.

Person-Centered Care

The physician William Osler once said, "It is important to know what disease the person has, but it is more important to know what person the disease has." A retired social worker newly diagnosed with Alzheimer's, expresses the same concept: "A person with Alzheimer's disease is many more things than just their diagnosis. Each person is a whole human being. It's important to be both sympathetic and curious and to have a real interest in discovering who that person is."[2] These two statements both speak to the core principle of an important movement called "person-centered care."

Person-centered care originated in the early 1990s in Great Britain through the work of the late Tom Kitwood, a social psychologist and founder of the Bradford School of Dementia Care. Kitwood taught that it is important for caregivers to understand the life history, personality, and communication style of a person with Alzheimer's in order to build respectful relationships and provide dignified care.[3] This is particularly important because, as your symptoms advance, it may be harder for you to share information with others about your background or your likes and dislikes. If someone doesn't know about you as a person, they may treat you like anyone else, and this depersonalizes and devalues their relationship with you. Person-centered care also emphasizes your remaining abilities rather than your losses and aims to create environments in which abilities can be realized and nurtured. Activities and schedules are adjusted to a person's unique temperament, interests, and needs, so residents can participate in the decisions that affect their daily well-being.

The Eden Alternative

In the United States, William Thomas, a Harvard-educated physician, pioneered the Eden Alternative as a means of deinstitutionalizing long-term care by incorporating more of the physical qualities, daily routines, and customs of a home environment. Gardens, welcoming interior spaces with inviting kitchens and comfortable recreation areas, resident pets, and involvement with the community, particularly with children, are essential features in residences modeled after the Eden Alternative. Research suggests that the Eden Alternative is improving quality of life and quality of care for long-term care residents. Staff also benefit from these humane, relationship-affirming practices and report greater satisfaction in their efforts to provide care. The Eden Alternative is also beginning to be taught to families who are caring for a loved one.

A "Best Friends" Approach to Alzheimer's Care

The Best Friends Approach has gained momentum in the United States and Canada. This movement originated with the work of Virginia Bell, a social worker, and David Troxel, a public health and Alzheimer's specialist, who advocate that the ingredients of quality care for people with Alzheimer's can be based on the principles of being a best friend. This down-to-earth approach teaches professional and family care partners to develop the "knack"—a set of relationship skills in "the art of doing difficult things with ease" that include ways to be supportive, loving, and empathic to the feelings of the person with Alzheimer's in order to foster a sense of value and safety.[4]

Historically, care has focused on the "patient" being taken care of by someone else in a position of authority. The Best Friends Approach advocates for greater partnership and relationship between parties and nurtures the tremendous importance of friendship and connection. Treat a person with Alzheimer's with the same care you would afford a best friend, and this seemingly simple approach can have profoundly beneficial consequences.

The principles of these care practices and organizations may seem like common sense in providing good care, and yet they cannot be taken for granted. These relatively new approaches are transforming the way Alzheimer's services and long-term care are practiced and hold promise in affording greater dignity and respectful care to people with Alzheimer's throughout life.

The Growing Field of Assistive Technology

We are all, for better or for worse, becoming ever more reliant on technology, and these advances may have helpful and creative applications in affording people with Alzheimer's greater independence. Some people with early-stage Alzheimer's are already beginning to rely on helpful technologies to adapt to memory loss or maximize functioning. For example:

- Voice-activated computers write dictated information so you don't have to type.
- Voice-activated cell phones call a person for you on command so you don't need to remember phone numbers or push buttons. More people are also carrying cell phones, so loved ones can track them down if needed.
- Medication dispensers organize daily pills and provide voice alarms that tell the person with memory loss to take their medicine.
- Pocket-sized global positioning systems may help a person find their way home when out on a walk.

- Computer-generated email, cognitive stimulation programs, video sports, and others educational programs are being used by people with early-stage Alzheimer's for communication and recreation.

As the population ages, and the technologically oriented Baby Boom Generation advances toward greater risk of developing Alzheimer's, many different industries are clamoring to find innovative ways to maximize independent living. Technology industries are partnering with heathcare industries to develop systems that will better allow people with Alzheimer's to more effectively manage memory loss in the home. For example, telephones may be equipped with visual aids that show you a picture of who is calling along with the person's name, relationship to you, and key facts about them and your last conversation to prompt your memory. "Smart Homes" might employ sensing systems to manage the home and alert you to turn off a light, close the refrigerator door, or turn off a faucet.

Other technologies may allow loved ones to better communicate with you or track your well-being when you're alone at home. Webcam systems (a camera used with a computer to transmit live images) hooked up between your home and a technology-savvy son or daughter can allow you to see one another and to interact via the computer screen. In the future, sensors placed throughout the home could notify loved ones of whether you have gone to bed, if you walked out the front door late at night, if you are at the stove cooking, or if you have fallen. While this kind of technology sounds intrusive or too futuristic to some, others welcome the idea of greater independence at home and the security of knowing that others could look out for them or be in closer communication without having to be physically present.

In all of the focus on finding a cure, it is easy to overlook the strides we have made in treatment of people with Alzheimer's and the ways we continue to strive to improve that care. But perhaps most importantly, never underestimate the progress that is made in homes each day, where families are trying their best to continue learning and loving as they make their own progress through the challenges of daily living. Those are often the advances that have the greatest impact and deserve the most grateful acknowledgment.

Questions for Discussion

- Are you currently taking any medication to treat Alzheimer's? If so, do you think it is helping?
- Do you have any concerns about future care needs? If so, what are they?
- Do you make use of any technology to help you manage memory loss?

Suggestions for Effective Participation in Your Treatment and Care

- Make every effort to take care of your physical health through regular exercise and healthy diet.
- Notify your doctor of any sudden changes in your symptoms or mood that could be due to another treatable medical condition.
- Consider ways that technology might help you manage memory loss and begin to use new cell phones, computer software, or other devices. It may take awhile to learn to use new technology, and repetition and routine use will be helpful.

Chapter Twenty-Nine

Complementary and Alternative Therapies

The National Center for Complementary and Alternative Medicine defines complementary and alternative medicine as "a group of diverse medical and healthcare systems, practices, and products, that are not currently part of conventional medicine." For people living in Western industrialized countries, many of these alternative practices have their origins in ancient Eastern cultures, where they may have been practiced for thousands of years. Complementary therapies can also include use of nutritional supplements or involvement in various practices aimed at physical or emotional well-being. This chapter provides a brief overview of the complementary and alternative therapies most commonly discussed in the treatment of Alzheimer's and related disorders.

> *It is important to inform your doctor of any complementary therapies you are using or exploring.*

Should I Take Any Vitamin or Mineral Supplements?

There has been considerable research into the effectiveness of various vitamins and minerals in the treatment of Alzheimer's. Vitamins E and C are antioxidants and have been investigated for their possible benefits to brain cells (see Chapter 21). A large, federally funded study that evaluated the effectiveness of 2,000 IUs of vitamin E per day in people with Alzheimer's found a small benefit to people with advanced Alzheimer's. However, more recent studies have revealed that there may be serious risks associated with high doses of vitamin E, particularly in people with heart disease, and high doses of vitamin E are no longer routinely recommended for Alzheimer's treatment. Blood levels of vitamin C have been found to be lower in some persons with Alzheimer's, but research has not confirmed a benefit to high doses of vitamin C in the management of Alzheimer's symptoms or progression.

Vitamins B12, and Folate (Folic Acid) have been investigated for their influence in Alzheimer's. Vitamin B12 deficiency can produce symptoms of dementia, and treatment of vitamin B12 deficiency is essential in any physician's evaluation of memory loss. Folate levels can also be low in people with Alzheimer's. Folate and vitamin B12 both help to regulate homocysteine, a chemical in the body that is elevated in many people with Alzheimer's. A large clinical trial to evaluate the benefit of B12, B6, and folate supplements in people with Alzheimer's who were not vitamin deficient concluded that while supplements of these vitamins did decrease homocysteine levels, B vitamins did not affect the symptoms or course of the disease. Although B vitamins may be beneficial for other conditions, they are not an effective treatment for Alzheimer's.

Numerous claims are made about the benefits of a variety of minerals for people who have Alzheimer's, including selenium and zinc. There is no evidence that mineral supplements are helpful in treating Alzheimer's, and minerals may actually be harmful in high doses. Although research findings from investigations into various vitamins and minerals has not been promising for Alzheimer's treatment, there may be other health benefits to these supplements in the management of other conditions. It is important to remember, however, that more is not always better with vitamins and minerals, and any use of these supplements should be discussed with your doctor.

Making Sense of Nutritional and Herbal Supplements

Omega fatty acids, specifically DHA, have received considerable attention for their benefits to healthy heart function. DHA also plays a role in healthy brain membrane function and is particularly important to the developing brain during infancy and childhood. DHA has been studied as a treatment for Alzheimer's, but high doses (equivalent to one to two helpings of fish per day) were not found to improve symptoms or slow the rate of change in study participants with Alzheimer's. DHA could conceivably play a role in the prevention of Alzheimer's, however, and there will likely be further studies to evaluate its protective benefits.

CoenzymeQ10 is produced by the human body and is important for the healthy function of cells. It is also an antioxidant that has been marketed as beneficial to the brain. However, there is no evidence of its effectiveness in treating or preventing Alzheimer's. A synthetic version of coenzyme Q10, called Idebenone, was tested in large clinical trials for the treatment of Alzheimer's, but the trials were stopped due to lack of benefit.

Ginkgo biloba is extracted from the leaf of the ginkgo tree and has been widely studied for its touted benefits to memory and thinking abilities. It is marketed for brain health due to its antioxidant and anti-inflammatory properties and other possible benefits to cells and brain chemicals. While some studies found that persons with Alzheimer's showed mild improvement with use of gingko biloba, the improvement was generally no better than placebo and is not as significant as that seen with the medications currently approved for Alzheimer's treatment. Ginkgo biloba may have an effect on blood clotting, so it is important to consult with your physician before taking this supplement.

Huperzine A is also marketed in health food stores for brain health. The compound is derived from a Chinese moss, and there is some scientific evidence that it can have a beneficial impact on many aspects of brain function. Findings from a large federally funded clinical trial of Huperzine A conducted in the United States suggest that the herb could improve some symptoms of Alzheimer's much like currently approved Alzheimer's medications.

Further study is warranted, however, to determine whether these beneficial effects are sufficient enough to warrant recommendation of this herb for people with Alzheimer's. Although Huperzine A was well tolerated in clinical trials, a physician should monitor any personal use of Huperzine A to identify any possible ill side effects.

The Booming Business of "Brain Boosters"

There are countless supplements and nutritional drinks that claim to stimulate thinking abilities, help prevent Alzheimer's, or boost brainpower. While some consumers may derive a perceived benefit from a particular supplement, to date, there is limited scientific evidence that any marketed brain booster can significantly alter the course or symptoms of Alzheimer's, let alone provide a cure. Many brain-booster elixirs are a mixture of vitamins, herbs, and other substances or compounds, such as omega fatty acids, that have been studied individually without promising results. It is unclear whether a combination of these compounds taken together can produce a more encouraging outcome, but supplements can be expensive and consumer caution is warranted.

The Food and Drug Administration (FDA) does not review data on the effectiveness of nutritional supplements or "nutraceuticals." The manufacturers of nutritional supplements are not required to provide the FDA with any evidence of a product's safety or ability to provide significant treatment. Thus, consumers may be enticed by the effective marketing of unwarranted claims based on little or no research. The purity or potency of supplements can also vary considerably among manufacturing brands, and there is currently no scientifically based recommended dose of these supplements for people with Alzheimer's. Many people assume that if something is "natural," it can't be harmful, but some supplements do have side effects or interactions with other medications that could compromise your health.

A product may also be marketed as a "medical food," meaning that it requires a prescription from a doctor. The FDA does regulate medical foods to some extent for safety, but medical foods do not undergo the rigorous trials for efficacy that drugs do. For example, levels of glucose (an energy source) are reduced in the brains of people with Alzheimer's. A product called Axona, a powder mixed with water to make a beverage, aims to compensate for this reduction by providing an alternative source of energy to the brain. Other medical foods aimed at the treatment of Alzheimer's will likely become available in the near future, and you should consult with your doctor about any possible benefits of these products.

Individual response to supplements or medical foods can vary. You may be curious about touted benefits of certain products, or perhaps you have experienced a positive outcome from their use. The use of supplements is a personal decision, but it is important to inform your doctor or other health-care provider of any nutritional supplements you are taking.

The Myths of Metals

Some people may gravitate to nutritional supplements for positive effects on symptoms while others may seek to avoid certain compounds for fear their symptoms may worsen. Exposure to toxic levels of mercury and other metals can be harmful to the brain. This has led to concern about commonly used dental fillings that are made of a mixture of metals, including mercury, and some health advocates suggest removing metal fillings in people with Alzheimer's. There have been a number of thorough and reputable studies examining any relationship between dental fillings and Alzheimer's. Researchers have carefully concluded that metal-based dental fillings do not increase the risk for Alzheimer's, and there is certainly no evidence that removing them will alter symptoms or prevent progression in people who already have Alzheimer's.

Aluminum has also been the subject of ongoing controversy. Trace levels of aluminum (as well as other metals) can be found in the brains of people with Alzheimer's at the time of death. This has led to concern about exposure to aluminum through everyday sources such as pots and pans, beverage cans, antacids, and antiperspirants. Numerous studies have failed to confirm any role of aluminum in causing Alzheimer's, and few scientists today believe that everyday sources of aluminum pose a threat or have any impact on symptoms or progression.

Due to concern about the effects of toxic amounts of metals and minerals on the brain, some alternative health practitioners have advocated chelation therapy for people with Alzheimer's. Chelation is a process whereby metals are removed from the bloodstream. Although some preliminary Alzheimer's research has explored means of removing metal deposits in the brain, there is no evidence that chelation therapy as currently practiced is a safe or effective treatment.

The Practices of Aromatherapy and Acupuncture

Aromatherapy is the therapeutic use of essential oils derived specifically from herbs or other plant materials. There is historic evidence of the use of aromatherapy in ancient civilizations including Egypt, Greece, and China. Essential oils produce scents that are thought to have beneficial effects, usually to one's emotional well-being. One theory is that the smelling of certain scents sends chemical messages to the limbic system, the region of the brain most responsible for our mood and emotions. The limbic system is linked to many other regions of the brain that affect overall physiological health. Many people with Alzheimer's have a reduced sense of smell, but certain chemicals in essential oils may be absorbed through the lungs during inhalation and then make their way to the brain. Essential oils are also absorbed through the skin when applied in lotions or other topical treatments.

Essential oils are used in skin and bath products, sprays, candles, oil lamps, and diffusers. Aromatherapy (specifically the essential oil of lavender) has been used for its perceived calming effects. Although there is limited scientific evidence of the efficacy of aromatherapy, there are no significant side effects, and an increasing number of long-term care homes are experimenting with aromatherapy to improve the well-being of their residents. Essential oils should never be ingested or applied topically undiluted, but they can be enjoyed in a lotion massaged into the skin or through scents released into the air, such as in the bedroom to promote sleep.

The practice of acupuncture originated in China. It involves temporarily inserting fine needles (usually not painful or even detected by the patient) into the skin at various places in an attempt to unblock or balance the flow of energy (called "chi" or "qi") throughout the body. In recent decades, acupuncture has been incorporated into some Western medicine practices and is most often used for pain management. There is increased investigation into the benefits of acupuncture for numerous other emotional and physical health conditions, but at present, there is no evidence that acupuncture can treat the progression or symptoms of Alzheimer's.

Therapies Involving the Creative Arts

Therapies involving the creative arts are not designed to cure symptoms or slow the rate of change in Alzheimer's. Rather, their therapeutic value lies in providing a meaningful activity that can stimulate thinking and attention, promote verbal or non-verbal expression, and help improve mood and quality of life. Many people may dismiss involvement in the arts due to concerns about lack of creativity or ability. Yet these activities can be particularly beneficial to people with no previous background in the arts because they don't harbor expectations about their creative performance. While some previously accomplished artists, musicians, or writers with Alzheimer's continue to enjoy their creative process and even use it to document their current experiences, others are hard on themselves when symptoms interfere with previously valued skills, and may turn away from their creative practice entirely. Participation in creative arts processes is a personal decision, but it rarely hurts to give available programs a try, as they may offer meaningful benefits.

Memories in the Making is a nationwide art program specially designed for people with Alzheimer's that is sponsored by Alzheimer's Association chapters and other organizations throughout the country. Using various art media, participants are encouraged to communicate their thoughts and feelings through painting and drawing. Experienced artists work with groups or individuals in various community settings using techniques that foster self-esteem and creative verbal and non-verbal communication. ARTZ: Artists for Alzheimer's is another example of an innovative program aimed at bringing art into the lives of people with Alzheimer's. Volunteers and staff in the various components of this international program engage people with Alzheimer's in the arts through direct creative expression or through specially designed museum tours developed for families facing Alzheimer's so they can enjoy a variety of cultural institutions together.

For many people, music provides enjoyment throughout life. Music can be energizing, calming, intellectually stimulating, or emotionally moving. For people with Alzheimer's, music can stimulate therapeutic movement and evoke memories that may otherwise be dormant or less accessible due to the onset of memory loss. Other creative arts include writing groups, theatre, or story telling. For example, TimeSlips, developed by Anne Basting, PhD, includes group process to engage people with Alzheimer's or a related disorder in storytelling that focuses less on the need to recall memories and more on the enduring ability of imagination.

Many people find that creative expression and accessing memories through the arts is an enjoyable experience, but not all memories and the emotions associated with them are positive. A particular piece of music or a work of art may take you back to a challenging time or a moment that is best left forgotten. It is important to be aware of all of the varied thoughts, feelings, or memories that creative expression evokes. Share your responses with others as a way to stimulate your attention and memory, and acknowledge any emotional responses.

Questions for Discussion

- Have you used any alternative or complementary therapies? If so, what was your experience?
- Have you explored any creative arts since the onset of Alzheimer's? If so, what was your experience?
- Have you heard of other alternative or complementary treatments not discussed in this chapter?

- Are you comfortable talking with your doctor about your use of any alternative or complementary therapies? If not, what is your concern?

Suggestions for Being an Informed Consumer of Alternative or Complementary Therapies

- Investigate the treatment claims of any therapy before you make use of it.
- Talk with your doctor or check this resource to help determine whether the claims are reasonable or legitimate: National Center for Complementary and Alternative Medicine at 888-644-6226 or www.nccam.nih.gov.
- Check with your insurance to determine whether it will cover any complementary therapies. Unfortunately, most complementary therapies are not covered for treatment of Alzheimer's.
- Buy any supplements from well-regarded pharmacies or health food stores where staff are knowledgeable about the origins and quality of their products.
- When seeking expressive arts therapies, determine whether the practitioner has experience working with people with Alzheimer's and is comfortable working with your memory loss or other symptoms.

Chapter Thirty

Research Brings Hope for the Future

Alzheimer's Disease International estimates that more than 35 million people worldwide will have Alzheimer's or a related disorder in 2010, and this growing number poses an international concern. Scientists around the world are working collaboratively (and often competitively!) to make progress in the evaluation, treatment, and prevention of these conditions. The last few decades have witnessed exciting and rapidly developing advances in these core areas, and the momentum continues to build as researchers explore promising new avenues of study.

> *"Participating in research gives me hope and assurance that I am doing all that I can do."*

Improving Methods for Early Detection and Accurate Diagnosis

Through sophisticated methods of brain imaging (taking pictures of the brain) researchers are gaining the tools to make a more certain diagnosis of Alzheimer's at earlier stages in the illness, and to distinguish it from other related disorders. Promising methods of brain imaging include types of Magnetic Resonance Imaging (MRI) as well as Positron Emission Tomography (PET). Scientists think that changes in the brain may begin many years before Alzheimer's symptoms become apparent. Brain imaging, as well as measurements of certain protein levels in cerebrospinal fluid (obtained through a lumbar puncture), may help to detect the earliest possible changes that suggest Alzheimer's onset. Certain neuropsychological measures (tests of memory and other areas of thinking) and functional assessments (changes in daily ability) may also help detect important early changes and help to differentiate normal changes that come with aging from more worrisome ones associated with the beginning of a dementia. Researchers are also exploring whether earlier detection of these physical and cognitive changes may allow for possible new treatments to be administered that could prevent or postpone development of symptoms.

Exploring New Pathways for Treatment

Many scientists believe that the likely cause of Alzheimer's is the body's abnormal processing of beta-amyloid protein into fragments that form sticky plaques in the brain. There are many areas of research aimed at stopping this destructive process with the hope that it will prevent Alzheimer's progression. Some studies are investigating whether a vaccine can be effective in immunizing people with Alzheimer's against beta-amyloid's damaging effects, while other researchers are exploring methods of blocking gamma secretase, an enzyme that helps create beta-amyloid. Some scientists are interested in the role of tau protein in the destruction of brain cells, and treatments may also be developed that specifically target the effects of this protein.

Investigation into the benefits of nerve growth factor (a substance produced in the brain to help cells work effectively), is underway in the hope that it can be administered directly into the brain to prevent cell death and slow the progression of Alzheimer's. Meanwhile, researchers are only beginning to explore the potential of stem cells in the treatment of

Alzheimer's, and this area of research will likely receive much more atten-tion in the coming years.

Researchers also continue to explore the possible benefits of various antioxidant and anti-inflammatory compounds, hoping that they can rem-edy some of the brain inflammation and cell damage that accompanies Alzheimer's. Many scientists believe that treatment for Alzheimer's may ulti-mately include a combination of therapies that work together to maintain levels of critical neurotransmitters in the brain, reduce the production of beta-amyloid protein, improve overall nerve cell health, and limit cell death. While it may be difficult to cure Alzheimer's once it has reached a certain stage, researchers hope that they can considerably slow down disease pro-gression and arrest symptoms at an early stage.

Working Toward Alzheimer's Prevention

Many people with Alzheimer's want to know how their children or loved ones can reduce their risk of developing the disease. Prevention is a very active area of research. Scientists believe that cardiovascular disease and dia-betes prevention are important, as are the roles of diet, exercise, and ongo-ing social and cognitive stimulation in Alzheimer's prevention. Specifically, maintaining good circulation to the brain with moderate exercise has been repeatedly shown to be helpful.

One can maintain a healthy lifestyle and do all of the right things to pro-mote physical and emotional well-being and still be vulnerable to the onset of any number of disabilities or unexpected challenges throughout life. Future generations can try to prevent the onset of Alzheimer's symptoms, and they may indeed be successful. But that will not eliminate any number of other vulnerabilities of growing older. Perhaps what is equally important in our attempts to prevent Alzheimer's and related disorders is the work being done to prevent the fear, stigma, and isolation that can accompany these con-ditions. Everyone living with Alzheimer's and anyone at risk for developing any kind of disability must be empowered with the information, resources, and emotional support needed to live a dignified and meaningful life.

Gaining Greater Understanding of the Alzheimer's Experience

Many people associate research with laboratories and science experiments, but there are many researchers working to better understand how to help families live a meaningful and good quality of life in the face of Alzheimer's. Researchers explore the effectiveness of socially and mentally stimulating programs for people with Alzheimer's and their families, educational interventions for care partners, methods of coping, and they may conduct interviews with individuals with Alzheimer's or their loved ones to better understand their experiences and feelings. All of this research aims to help sensitize professionals and the public to the needs of families while also providing helpful evaluation of attempts to provide care.

There has been growing interest in better understanding what it is like to have Alzheimer's, and this body of research is obviously not possible without the partnership of people with Alzheimer's who are willing to share their thoughts and feelings with others. Elaine Robinson, who has young-onset Alzheimer's, writes:

> "I really think that people like myself should be encouraged to take part in research and made to feel that their contributions, no matter how small, would be greatly valued. After all, who else would know what it's like to have this disease?....What a hugely missed opportunity it would be if people with Alzheimer's were excluded from the very thing that could be used to gain a fuller understanding of their disease."[1]

Participating in Research

Research advances rely on volunteers who have Alzheimer's, their care partners, and family members or concerned others who do not have symptoms but may be at future risk. Although the majority of people with Alzheimer's may never participate in research, for those who do, it can be a rewarding and meaningful experience. Victor Dimeo writes:

"Why not share anything I learn in Alzheimer's and help people to work with it and learn from it? There is much work being done throughout the world with research studies. There is hope that a solution will soon be forthcoming. I would like to take part in the cure. I feel that I can live longer by participating in research. Leave something of yourself for the world so that you can participate in its future."[2]

One significant way that people with Alzheimer's can participate in research and have an impact on the future is through enrollment in a clinical trial. Clinical trials are worldwide and are essential to advancing progress in many areas of Alzheimer's research.

Understanding Clinical Trials

A clinical trial is the study of a drug, procedure, or device aimed at improving the diagnosis, treatment, or prevention of a medical condition. Clinical trials occur in three phases before any new medication, procedure, or treatment is approved by the Food and Drug Administration (FDA).

Phase 1 trials enroll small groups of people to evaluate the overall safety or side effects of a drug or procedure and to establish appropriate drug dosage. Studies have usually been conducted in animal models before they reach Phase 1 human trials. In Phase 2 trials, the drug or treatment is given to a larger group of people evaluate its effectiveness and to further monitor its safety. If Phase 2 trials are promising, the project moves into a Phase 3 trial. These trials usually involve even higher numbers of participants and last longer than the previous trials. Their aim is to further validate the effectiveness and safety of the treatment and possibly compare the treatment with any standard therapy currently being used. At the end of Phase 3 trials, the FDA has usually collected enough data to determine whether the drug under investigation is safe and beneficial enough to warrant approval.

Clinical trials for experimental drugs or procedures have various designs, but usually the most scientifically respected design is a "placebo-controlled double-blind study." A placebo is a compound that looks like the one under investigation, but it has no active ingredients. Up to half of the participants in these kinds of studies receive a placebo. This allows the researchers to compare those who receive treatment with those who do not and ensures greater confidence in the trial outcomes. Some people do not want to participate in a clinical trial if there is a chance of receiving a placebo. It is well documented, however, that people who are unknowingly taking the placebo can experience symptom improvement simply because they believe they could be taking something beneficial. "Double blind" means that neither you nor the researchers in charge of the clinical trial know whether you are receiving the treatment or the placebo. This ensures that the researchers are unbiased during the trial and don't interpret or report findings influenced by their own hopes or objectives. Most Alzheimer's trials now incorporate a cross-over phase, so that even the subjects who are started in the placebo arm, are switched, after some period of time, to the treatment arm and have the opportunity to receive any benefits.

Am I Eligible for a Clinical Trial?

All clinical trials have inclusion and exclusion criteria. These criteria are based on your age, health status and history, and other medications you may already be taking that could interfere with the drug or procedure under investigation. If you do not qualify for one trial, you may qualify for a different one, and with rapid advances in Alzheimer's research, there are always new trials underway. Unfortunately, most clinical trials for Alzheimer's exclude participants under age 50 or 55, which is frustrating and disappointing for some people with young-onset Alzheimer's.

Enrolling in a clinical trial requires a study partner. This person ensures that you get to your appointments and that you take the treatment under investigation as directed. Ideally this study partner lives with you or, at minimum, has routine contact with you. Although the clinical trial team will be evaluating the effectiveness of any treatment with you during study visits, they also rely on your study partner to provide feedback about any positive or negative effects witnessed during your participation.

What Should I Know Before Enrolling in a Clinical Trial?

Before enrolling in a clinical trial, you should have ample opportunity to have all of your questions answered. You need to have a general understanding of what is required of you during the study and knowledge of the possible risks and benefits so that you can provide your "informed consent" to participate. The following questions may help you obtain the information you need before enrolling in a clinical trial:

- What is the name of the drug or procedure being studied?
- What are the hoped-for benefits of the drug or procedure under investigation?
- Are there possible negative side effects?
- What are my chances of being on placebo versus the active treatment?
- Will I receive the active treatment at any point during or after the study?
- Will participation in this clinical trial exclude me from participating in other trials in the future?
- What is the time commitment, including total length of the clinical trial and the number and duration of visits?
- Are there any medical procedures involved in participation, such as a blood draw, brain scan, or lumbar puncture?
- Is there any cost to participating? Who covers any medical expenses incurred during the trial?

Your participation in a clinical trial must be voluntary, with the understanding that you can withdraw from the study if necessary. Although participation requires time and commitment from both you and your study partner, many participants report positive benefits from the support and attention derived from repeated visits with the clinical trial team.

You Can Make a Difference

Since most studies only allow people in the early to middle stages of Alzheimer's to participate, it is important to be proactive and seek out hopeful clinical trials before symptoms advance. Participation in clinical trials can be rewarding for you and your family, and for the benefit of future generations. All of the currently approved treatments for Alzheimer's would not be available now without the volunteers who participated in the clinical trials. Bernie Shapiro writes in an Alzheimer's Association newsletter:

> "After the initial shock of the diagnosis, and the realization that our lives would be changing in ways we had not anticipated, we took stock of our lives. We would learn as much as we could and seek ways to gain quality time and life. We explored options for treatment and became very interested in research programs. Barbara and I realize that medicine and science are the direct result of new ideas and approaches developed through research. It is important to realize that without knowledge, we stumble into darkness. I am participating in a number of research programs. Hopefully they will be of some help to me, but if not, I am confident that they will benefit others in the years to come. Participating in research gives me hope and assurance that I am doing all that I can do."[3]

Questions for Discussion

- Have you heard about any exciting Alzheimer's research in the news? Have you been able to get answers to any questions you have about possible Alzheimer's treatments?
- Would you be interested in participating in research? Why or why not?
- Have you ever participated in a clinical trial? If so, what was your experience?

Suggestions for Finding Out More about Research and Clinical Trials

- Cut out articles about Alzheimer's research that you see in newspapers or magazines so you can ask your doctor or local Alzheimer's organizations any questions you have about the information.

- Although you have already been diagnosed, it cannot hurt to follow Alzheimer's prevention guidelines to afford yourself any extra benefits to maintaining brain health.
- If you would like to participate in research or learn more about clinical trials and other hopeful areas of investigation and study, contact:
  – Alzheimer's Disease Centers, funded by the National Institutes on Aging, are located around the country. Call ADEAR at 800-438-4380 or find research center locations at www.nia.nih.gov/Alzheimers/ResearchInformation/ResearchCenters.
  – Alzheimer's Disease Cooperative Study at www.adcs.org.
  – Fisher Center for Alzheimer's Research Foundation at 800-259-4636 or www.alzinfo.org.
  – Clinical Trials.Gov is a service of the National Institutes of Health at www.clinicaltrials.gov.

Helpful Resources

The following is a condensed listing of major national and international organizations serving people with Alzheimer's disease and related disorders that may be of assistance to you and your loved ones. Many other organizations and resources are referenced throughout this book as they relate to specific chapter topics.

Alzheimer's Association
800-272-3900
www.alz.org
The Alzheimer's Association is headquartered in Chicago with regional chapters throughout the United States. They maintain a 24-hour helpline, are active in advocacy and research, and maintain a number of core services and programs for families facing Alzheimer's through their chapters. They have a section on their Web site specifically for people with Alzheimer's as well as a message board for communicating with others.

Alzheimer's Disease Education and Referral (ADEAR)
800-438-4380
http://www.nia.nih.gov/alzheimers
ADEAR is a service of the National Institute on Aging. They provide extensive and reliable information on Alzheimer's and related disorders. Many of their excellent publications are available to download from their Web site. They also list Alzheimer's Research Centers across the country as well as current clinical trials.

Alzheimer's Foundation of America (AFA)
866-232-8484
www.alzfdn.org
AFA is a consortium of more than 1200 member organizations across the country dedicated to improving the care of families facing Alzheimer's. The foundation's headquarters is based in New York, where it organizes national educational, advocacy, and information and referral services for families facing Alzheimer's.

Alzheimer's Disease International (ADI)

www.alz.co.uk

ADI is an umbrella organization of worldwide Alzheimer organizations. ADI networks with international chapters, encourages research, supports an annual international conference, and provides information to families facing Alzheimer's. Their Web site has a section, "I Have Dementia" that provides helpful information and resources.

Alzheimer Society of Canada

www.alzheimer.ca

The Alzheimer Society of Canada maintains an excellent section of their national Web site called "I Have Alzheimer's Disease" for people with Alzheimer's or a related dementia that includes valuable information, interactive opportunities, upcoming events, and resources.

Alzheimer Europe

www.alzheimer-europe.org

Alzheimer Europe is an umbrella organization of Alzheimer associations from 30 countries across Europe. Their Web site has a comprehensive category called "Living with Dementia" that provides helpful information to individuals and families facing Alzheimer's or a related disorder.

Alzheimer's Society

www.alzheimers.org.uk

The Alzheimer's Society serves England, Wales, and Northern Ireland. Their Web site has a section called "Talking Point" that offers opportunities for people with Alzheimer's and their families to network.

Alzheimer Scotland

www.alzscot.org

This Web site includes a valuable section called "For People with Dementia" that includes a great deal of practical information and personal testimony from people with Alzheimer's and related disorders.

Alzheimer's Australia

www.fightdementia.org.au
See this Web site under the heading "I Have Dementia" for a series of helpful fact sheets written for persons with Alzheimer's or a related disorder on a variety of topics.

Alzheimer's New Zealand

www.alzheimers.org.nz
This Web site provides useful information for people with Alzheimer's on a variety of topics under the heading "Help and Support."

Dementia Advocacy and Support Network International (DASNI)

www.dasninternational.org
DASNI is an international Internet-based support network organized by and for people with Alzheimer's or a related dementia. The organization provides opportunities for online chat rooms as well as other networking and advocacy opportunities.

Association for Frontotemporal Degeneration

866-507-7222
www.theaftd.org
This national organization aims to fund research as well as provide information, education, and support to families facing a frontotemporal dementia. The Web site includes resources and support services for families in the United States and Canada.

Lewy Body Dementia Association

800-539-9767
www.lewybodydementia.org
This comprehensive Web site provides information, resources and networking opportunities for families facing dementia with Lewy bodies or Parkinson's disease with dementia.

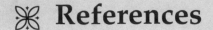# ✼ References

Chapter 1: What Is Alzheimer's Disease?

1. *Contexts – A Forum for the Medical Humanities*, The Institute for Medicine in Contemporary Society at the University at Stony Brook, New York 8, no 3 (2000): 11.
2. *Principles for a Dignified Diagnosis*, Chicago, IL: Alzheimer's Association, 2009. *Principles for a Dignified Diagnosis* is available to view and print at http://www.alz.org.

Chapter 2: Understanding Your Reactions to the Diagnosis

1. J. Anthony, "Ideas About Alzheimer's," Eastern Massachusetts Chapter of the Alzheimer's Association Summer/Fall 1997 newsletter.
2. L. Snyder, M.P Quayhagen, S. Shepherd, B. Bower, "Supportive seminar groups: an intervention for early stage dementia patients," *The Gerontologist* 35 (1995): 691-695.
3. *What Happens Next? – A booklet about being diagnosed with Alzheimer's disease or a related disorder*. National Institutes of Health Publication No: 07-6199, October, 2008: 5.
4. R. Davis, *My Journey Into Alzheimer's*, Wheaton, IL: Tyndale House Publishers, 1989: 91.
5. D. Tilleli, "Reflections," *Perspectives – A Newsletter for Individuals with Alzheimer's or a Related Disorder* 2, no. 3 (2007): 1-2.
6. J. Anthony, "Ideas About Alzheimer's," Eastern Massachusetts Chapter of the Alzheimer's Association Summer/Fall 1997 newsletter.
7. *"I Have Alzheimer's Disease" – A Chronicle of Human Experience*. A DVD of the Alzheimer Society of Belleville-Hastings-Quint, Ontario, Canada, 2005.
8. L. Snyder, *Speaking Our Minds- What it's Like to Have Alzheimer's (Revised Edition)*, Baltimore: Health Professions Press, 2009: 120.
9. L. Dennis, "Reducing Dread and Marginalization," *Perspectives* 16, no 4 (2001): 5.
10. B. Shapiro, "A Life Beyond the Diagnosis," *Massachusetts Chapter of the Alzheimer's Association Newsletter* 21, no. 4 (2003): 1, 4.

Chapter 3: Symptoms You Could Experience

1. O.A. Hoblitzelle, *The Majesty of Your Loving – A Couple's Journey Through Alzheimer's*, Cambridge MA: Green Mountain Books, 2008: 35.
2. D. Barlow, "A Communication Barrier," *Perspectives – A Newsletter for Individuals with Alzheimer's or a Related Disorder* 3, no 2 (1998): 6
3. The Early Stage Support Groups in the North/Central Okanagan Region of the Alzheimer Society of British Columbia, *Memory Problems?* Alzheimer Society of British Columbia, 2000: 5.
4. L. Snyder, *Speaking Our Minds – What it's Like to Have Alzheimer's (Revised Edition)*, Baltimore: Health Professions Press, 2009: 86
5. L. Snyder, *Speaking Our Minds – What it's Like to Have Alzheimer's*, 117
6. L. Snyder, M.P. Quayhagen, S. Shepherd, D. Bower, "Supportive seminar groups: An intervention for early stage dementia patients," *Gerontologist* 35, no 5 (1995): 694.
7. The Early Stage Support Groups in the North/Central Okanagan Region of the Alzheimer Society of B.C. *Memory Problems?* Alzheimer Society British Columbia, 2000: 4.
8. L. Snyder, *Speaking Our Minds – What it's Like to Have Alzheimer's*, 23.
9. A. Phinney, "Living with the Symptoms of Alzheimer's Disease." In P. Harris (Ed) *The Experience of Alzheimer's*, Baltimore: Johns Hopkins University Press, 2002: 56-57
10. P. Harris, "Intimacy, Sexuality, and Early-Stage Dementia–The Changing Marital Relationship," *Alzheimer's Care Today* 10, no 2 (2009): 69.

11. I. McLanathan, "Letter to the Editor," *Perspectives* 11, no 1 (2005): 5.

Chapter 4: Talking With Others About Having Alzheimer's

1. R. Bachrach, "Doing my best," *Perspectives – A Newsletter for Individuals with Alzheimer's or a Related Disorder* 3, no 1, (1997): 1
2. L. Snyder, *Speaking Our Minds – What it's Like to Have Alzheimer's (Revised Edition)*, Baltimore: Health Professions Press, 2009: 87.
3. V. Collins, "In My Own Voice," *Perspectives* 9, no 3 (2004): 2.
4. L. Snyder, "Disclosing the Diagnosis–Who and When to Tell," *Perspectives* 2, no 4 (1997):1.
5. L. Snyder, *Speaking Our Minds – What it's Like to Have Alzheimer's*, 69.
6. M. Gordon, "Letter to the Editor," *Perspectives* 13, no 4 (2008): 5.
7. L. Snyder, "Disclosing the Diagnosis–Who and When to Tell," *Perspectives* 2, no 4 (1997): 1.

Chapter 5: Taking Care of Family Relationships

1. *Enhancing Communication – An inspirational guide for people like us with early-stage memory loss. A By Us For Us Guide*, Waterloo, Ontario: Murray Alzheimer's Research and Education Program, University of Waterloo, 2008: 3.
2. P. Harris and G. Sterin, "Insider's perspective: Defining and preserving the self in dementia," *Journal of Mental Health and Aging* 5, no 3 (1999): 246.
3. L. Snyder, *Speaking Our Minds – What it's Like to Have Alzheimer's (Revised Edition)*. Baltimore: Health Professions Press, 2009: 103.
4. Alzheimer's Association, *Alzheimer's Disease Inside Looking Out*, A video production, Cleveland, OH: Cleveland Area Chapter, 1995.

Chapter 6: The Unique Concerns of Young-Onset Alzheimer's Families

1. L. Snyder, *Speaking Our Minds–What it's Like to Have Alzheimer's, (Revised Edition)* Baltimore: Health Professions Press, 2009: 142.
2. P. Harris, J. Keady, "Living with early onset dementia–Exploring the experience and developing evidence-based guidelines for practice," *Alzheimer's Care Quarterly* 5, no 2 (2004): 116.
3. P. Reed, S. Bluethmann, *Voices of Alzheimer's Disease–A Summary Report on the Nationwide Town Hall Meetings for People with Early Stage Dementia*, Chicago, IL: Alzheimer's Association, 2008: 9.
4. P. Reed, S. Bluethmann, *Voices of Alzheimer's Disease*, 28.
5. L. Snyder, *Speaking Our Minds–What it's Like to Have Alzheimer's*, 44.
6. Anonymous, *The Unexpected Journey–A Blog About Living with Younger Onset Alzheimer's*, 2009, Alzheimer's Association San Diego and Imperial Chapter website at https://secure2.convio.net/adrdsd/site/SPageServer?pagename=younger_onset_blog.
7. L. Snyder, *Speaking Our Minds–What it's Like to Have Alzheimer's*, 48.
8. P. Reed, S. Bluethmann, *Voices of Alzheimer's Disease*, 25.
9. L. Snyder, *Speaking Our Minds–What it's Like to Have Alzheimer's*, 148.
10. C. Jackson, "The Changing Face of Alzheimer's," *Perspectives–A Newsletter for Individuals with Alzheimer's or a Related Disorder* 12, no 2 (2007): 6-7

Chapter 7: Maintaining Friendships and Creating New Ones

1. L. Snyder, "Finding Meaningful Activity," *Perspectives – A Newsletter for Individuals with Alzheimer's or a Related Disorder* 13, no 1 (2007): 2.
2. *"I Have Alzheimer's Disease"–A Chronicle of Human Experience*. A DVD of the Alzheimer Society of Belleville-Hastings-Quint, Ontario, Canada, 2005.

3. S. Camiel, "Thoughts on the Importance of Community," *Perspectives* 12, no 3 (2007): 1-2.

Chapter 8: Strategies For Effective Communication with Friends and Family

1. D. Barlow, "A Communication Barrier," *Perspectives – A Newsletter for Individuals with Alzheimer's or a Related Disorder* 3, no 2 (1998): 6.
2. *Enhancing Wellness – An inspirational guide for people like us with early-stage memory loss. A By Us For Us Guide,* Waterloo, Ontario: Murray Alzheimer's Research and Education Program, University of Waterloo, 2008: 8.
3. C. Henderson, *Partial View: An Alzheimer's Journal,* Dallas: Southern Methodist University Press, 1998: 18.
4. M. Trabert, "The DRC Club." *Perspectives* 2, no 3 (1997): 7.
5. *Enhancing Communication – An inspirational guide for people like us with early-stage memory loss. A By Us For Us Guide,* Waterloo, Ontario: Murray Alzheimer's Research and Education Program, University of Waterloo, 2008: 89.
6. P. Reed, S. Bluethmann, *Voices of Alzheimer's Disease, A Summary Report on the Nationwide Town Hall Meetings for People with Early Stage Dementia.* Chicago, IL: Alzheimer's Association, 2008: 22.
7. Alzheimer's Association, *Alzheimer's Disease: Inside Looking Out.* A video production. Cleveland, OH: Cleveland Area Chapter, 1995.
8. K. Vetor, "Coffee House," *Early Alzheimer's–An International Newsletter on Dementia* 5, no 2 (2003): 9.

Chapter 9: Helpful Tips for Managing Memory Loss

1. Sheila, "What it's like to live with Alzheimer's." *Perspectives – A Newsletter for Individuals with Alzheimer's or a Related Disorder* 4, no 3 (1999): 1-3.
2. Sheila, *Perspectives,* 1-3.
3. L. Snyder, "A conversation with Bobby," *Perspectives* 3, no 3 (1998): 7.

Chapter 10: Dealing Effectively with Other Symptoms

1. C. Henderson, *Partial View: An Alzheimer's Journal.* Dallas: Southern Methodist University Press. 1998: 79.

Chapter 11: Improving the Safety of Your Home Environment

1. "Brainstorming," *Perspectives – A Newsletter for Individuals with Alzheimer's or a Related Disorder* 13, no 3 (2008): 7.

Chapter 12: Making Decisions About Driving

1. L. Snyder, *Speaking Our Minds – What it's Like to Have Alzheimer's (Revised Edition).* Baltimore: Health Professions Press, 2009: 66.
2. Anonymous, "To drive or not to drive," *Perspectives – A Newsletter for Individuals with Alzheimer's or a Related Disorder* 6, no 3 (2001): 6-7.
3. V. Collins, "In my own voice," *Perspectives* 9, no 3 (2004): 2.
4. L. Snyder, "A conversation with Bobby," *Perspectives* 3, no 3 (1998): 7.
5. C. LaBarge, "Living on my own with Alzheimer's," *Perspectives* 4, no 4 (1999): 2.
6. Anonymous, "To drive or not to drive," *Perspectives* 6, no 3 (2001) : 6-7. Alzheimer's Association, *The Emerging Voice of Alzheimer's.* A Web site for people in the early stages, 2009. Quote can be found at: http://www.alz.org/townhall/video06.asp.

Chapter 13: If You Live Alone

1. L. De Witt, J. Ploeg, M. Black, "Living on the threshold – the spatial experience of living alone with dementia," *Dementia* 8, no 2 (2009): 277.
2. L. Snyder, *Speaking Our Minds – What it's Like to Have Alzheimer's (Revised Edition)*, Baltimore: Health Professions Press, 2009: 71.
3. L Snyder, *Speaking Our Minds*, 76.

Chapter 14: Understanding and Managing Your Feelings

1. L. Snyder, *Speaking Our Minds – What it's Like to Have Alzheimer's (Revised Edition)*, Baltimore: Health Professions Press, 2009: 27.
2. Alzheimer's Association, *Alzheimer's Disease Inside Looking Out*. A video production. Cleveland, OH: Cleveland Area Chapter, 1995.
3. T. Raushi, "The Alzheimer's Survivor," *Perspectives – A Newsletter for Individuals with Alzheimer's or a Related Disorder* 7, no 4 (2002): 2.
4. L. Snyder, "What do we value about our support group?" *Perspectives* 6, no 3 (2001): 3.
5. D. Barlow, "A Communication Barrier," *Perspectives* 3, no 2 (1998): 7.
6. P.B. Harris, G.J. Sterin, "Insider's perspective: Defining and preserving the self in dementia," *Journal of Mental Health and Aging* 5, no 3 (1995): 241-256.
7. R. Simpson, A Simpson, *Through the Wilderness of Alzheimer's–A Guide in Two Voices*, Minneapolis: Augsburg Fortress, 1999: 79-80.
8. Alzheimer Society of Canada, *Speaking Out - Insights from People with Alzheimer's Disease*. Insert entitled, "Message to family and friends," Toronto, Ontario, 2002.
9. The Early Stage Support Groups in the North/Central Okanagan Region of the Alzheimer Society of B.C, *Memory Problems?* Alzheimer Society British Columbia, 2000: 6.
10. *What Happens Next? – A booklet about being diagnosed with Alzheimer's disease or a related disorder*, National Institutes of Health Publication No: 07-6199, October, 2008: 1.
11. L. Snyder, *Speaking Our Minds – What it's Like to Have Alzheimer's (Revised Edition)*, 77.
12. R. Davis, *My Journey Into Alzheimer's*, Wheaton, IL: Tyndale House, 1989: 109.
13. J. Killick, "Dark head amongst the grey: Experiencing the worlds of younger persons with dementia." In: S. Cox, J. Keady (eds), *Younger People with Dementia–Planning, Practice, and Development*, London and Philadelphia: Jessica Kingsley, 1999: 160.
14. R. Davis, *My Journey Into Alzheimer's*. Wheaton, IL: Tyndale House, 1989: 90.
15. L. Raymer, "An old lesson relearned," *Perspectives* 7, no 3 (2002): 6-7.
16. *Don't Make the Journey Alone – A Message from Fellow Travelers*, Alzheimer Scotland Action on Dementia. www.alzscot.org.
17. B. McNaughton, "Lost, Stolen, or Strayed," *Perspectives* 11, no 3 (2006): 2.
18. C. Edwards, J. Karlawish, "My new journey: One man's reflections on living with Alzheimer's disease," *The Quarterly – A Newsletter of the University of Pennsylvania*, Spring, 2006.
19. L. Snyder, *Speaking Our Minds – What it's Like to Have Alzheimer's (Revised Edition)*, 27.

Chapter 15: The Benefits of Support Groups For You and Your Family

1. C. Yeh-Gardner, T. Truscott, L. Snyder, "The benefits of support groups for persons with Alzheimer's disease," *Alzheimer's Care Quarterly* 2, no 4 (2001): 42-46.
2. S. Duff, "Alzheimer Scotland – action on dementia: younger person's group in Grampion, northeast Scotland," *Early Alzheimer's* 1, no 2 (1998): 4-5.
3. D. Morrow and Members of the Early-Stage Support Group in Montreal, Quebec, "Together: sharing the experiences of an early-stage support group," *Alzheimer Society of Montreal Newsletter*, Montreal, Quebec,

24, no 1, Spring 2006.

4. V. DiMeo, "Finding meaning in Alzheimer's." *Perspectives – A Newsletter for Individuals with Alzheimer's or a Related Disorder* 9, no 1 (2003): 2.

5. D. Morhardt, "Top 10 ideas for enhancing quality of life by diagnosed individuals and families living with Alzheimer's disease and related dementias," *Alzheimer's Care Quarterly* 5, no 2 (2004): 103-107.

6. Long Island Alzheimer's Foundation, "Early-stage client group – An introduction." *LIAFLine Newsletter of the Long Island Alzheimer's Foundation,* Port Washington: New York, January, 2006: 6.

7. L. Dennis, "A whole new me," *Perspectives* 8, no 2 (2002): 2.

Chapter 16: Learning to Accept Help When You Need It

1. L. De Witt, J. Ploeg, M. Black, "Living on the threshold – The spatial experience of living alone with dementia," *Dementia* 8, no 2 (2009): 279.

2. A. Rackley, S. Dembling, *I Can Still Laugh,* Dallas, Texas: University of Texas at Dallas Center for Brain Health, 2009: 93.

3. D. Seman, "Meaningful communication throughout the journey," In P. Harris (Ed.) *The Person with Alzheimer's Disease,* Baltimore: Health Professions Press, 2002: 144.

4. Snyder, L. *Speaking Our Minds – What it's Like to Have Alzheimer's (Revised Edition).* Baltimore: Health Professions Press, 2009: 71.

5. K.H. Zabbia, *Painted Diaries – A Mother and Daughter's Experience Through Alzheimer's.* Minneapolis: Fairview Press, 1996: 89.

6. *"I Have Alzheimer's Disease" – A Chronicle of Human Experience.* A DVD of the Alzheimer Society of Belleville-Hastings-Quint, Ontario, Canada, 2005.

7. H.E. Hedberg, "My father, my teacher, my future," *careADvantage - A Publication of the Alzheimer's Foundation of America,* Spring, 2008: 12-13.

Chapter 17: Finding Meaningful Activities

1. L. Snyder, "Activity and Alzheimer's: enhancing the quality of life," *Perspectives – A Newsletter for Individuals with Alzheimer's or a Related Disorder* 3, no 3 (1998): 1.

2. W. Deutsch, "I'm Still Me," *Early Alzheimer's – An International Newsletter on Dementia* 5, no 2 (2003): 11.

3. D. Morhardt, "Top 10 ideas for enhancing quality of life by diagnosed individuals and families living with Alzheimer's disease and related dementias," *Alzheimer's Care Quarterly* 5, no 2 (2004):103-107.

4. P. Michaud, "The importance of feeling connected," Alzheimer's Association New York City Newsletter, Fall, 2009. http://www.alznyc.org/nyc/newsletter/fall2009/05.asp.

5. M. Trabert, "An interview with Anne," *Perspectives* 6, no 2 (2006): 6.

6. L. Snyder, "Finding Meaningful Activity," *Perspectives* 13, no 1 (2007): 2.

7. L. Snyder, "Brainstorming," *Perspectives* 13, no 2 (2008): 4.

8. L. Snyder, "Brainstorming." *Perspectives* 13, no 3 (2008): 7.

9. Alzheimer's Association, *Alzheimer's Disease Inside Looking Out.* A video production. Cleveland, OH: Cleveland Area Chapter, 1995.

10. R. Bachrach, "Doing my best," *Perspectives* 3, no 1 (1997): 1.

Chapter 18: Speaking Your Mind Through Advocacy

1. V. DiMeo, "Finding meaning in Alzheimer's," *Perspectives – A Newsletter for Individuals with Alzheimer's or a Related Disorder* 9, no 1 (2003): 2.

2. Alzheimer's Association, *Sharing the Journey –Forging Relationships That Ease the Way,* New York: New York City Chapter, Disc 1 of DVD, April 20, 2005.

3. L. Snyder, "A Call to Action," *Perspectives* 11, no 1 (2005): 2.

4. B. Reisman, "Speaking out – A statement to congress from an Alzheimer's advocate." *Perspectives* 11, no 2

(2006): 6-7.

5. P. Reed, S. Bluethmann, *Voices of Alzheimer's Disease–A Summary Report on the Nationwide Town Hall Meetings for People with Early Stage Dementia.* Chicago, IL: Alzheimer's Association, 2008: 28.

6. L. Hogg, "Shedding the carapace" *Global Perspective–A Newsletter of Alzheimer's Disease International* 19, no 2 (September 2009): 10.

7. L. Drew, L. Ferrari, *Different Minds–Living with Alzheimer Disease.* New Brunswick: Goose Lane Editions, 2005: 7.

Chapter 20: The Benefits of Mental Stimulation

1. L. Snyder, M. Quayhagen, S. Shepherd, B. Bower, "Supportive seminar groups: an intervention for early stage dementia patients," *The Gerontologist* 35, no 5 (1995): 691-695.

2. Stanford Center on Longevity; Max Planck Institute for Human Development, "Expert consensus on brain health," 2009. http://longevity.stanford.edu/files/SCL_MPICogAging.pdf.

Chapter 21: Food for Thought: The Value of Good Nutrition

1 Reed, P, Bluethmann, S, *Voices of Alzheimer's Disease – A Summary Report on the Nationwide Town Hall Meetings for People with Early Stage Dementia,* Chicago, IL: Alzheimer's Association, 2008: 22.

Chapter 22: Maintaining Hope and a Sense of Humor

1. L. Snyder, "Family Relationships," *Perspectives – A Newsletter for Individuals with Alzheimer's or a Related Disorder* 7, no 3 (2002): 2.

2. Reed, P, Bluethmann, S. *Voices of Alzheimer's Disease – A Summary Report on the Nationwide Town Hall Meetings for People with Early Stage Dementia.* Chicago, IL: Alzheimer's Association, 2008: 19.

3. L. Snyder, "The Gift of Humor," *Perspectives* 1, no 4 (1996): 2-3.

4. P. Alderton, "Living positively with Alzheimer's disease," *Early Alzheimer's* 1, no 1 (1998): 5.

5. T. Raushi, "The Alzheimer's Survivor," *Perspectives* 7, no 4 (2002): 1.

6. R. Yale, L. Snyder, "The experience of support groups for persons with early-stage Alzheimer's and their families," In P. Harris (Ed), *The Experience of Alzheimer's,* Baltimore: Johns Hopkins University Press, 2002: 236.

7. L. Snyder, *Speaking Our Minds – What it's Like to Have Alzheimer's (Revised Edition),* Baltimore: Health Professions Press, 2009: 29.

8. Mayo Clinic, *Alzheimer's Disease: Voices From the Journey.* A video production of Mayo Clinic Alzheimer's Disease Research Center, Rochester, MN. 2000.

9. L. Snyder, *Speaking Our Minds – What it's Like to Have Alzheimer's (Revised Edition),* 53.

10. *Enhancing Wellness – An inspirational guide for people like us with early-stage memory loss - A By Us For Us Guide,* Waterloo, Ontario: Murray Alzheimer's Research and Education Program, University of Waterloo, 2008:10.

11. L. Snyder, "Satisfactions and challenges in spiritual faith and practice for persons with dementia," *Dementia* 2, no 3 (2003): 299-313.

12. E.L. Gorman, "Early stage support group: My step in the right direction?" *Perspectives* 16, no 4 (2001): 5.

13. L. Snyder, "Brainstorming," *Perspectives* 12, no 1 (2006): 6.

Chapter 23: Taking Care of Your Care Partner

1. E. Ballard, L. Gwyther, T.P. Toal, *Pressure Points – Alzheimer's and Anger,* North Carolina: Duke University Medical Group, 2000: 7.

2. L. Drew, L. Ferrari, *Different Minds – Living with Alzheimer Disease,* New Brunswick: Goose Lane Edi-

tions, 2005: 68.

3. R. Bachrach, "Doing my best," *Perspectives – A Newsletter for Individuals with Alzheimer's or a Related Disorder* 3, no 1 (1997): 2

4. L. Snyder, *Speaking Our Minds – What it's Like to Have Alzheimer's (Revised Edition)*, Baltimore: Health Professions Press, 2009: 25.

5. J. Fox, *I Still Do*, New York: Powerhouse Books, 2009: 35.

6. J. Tucker, "How to change 'surviving' into 'thriving.'" Rush Alzheimer's Disease Center newsletter. Chicago, IL: Rush Presbyterian St. Luke Medical Center, 1995.

7. L. Snyder, "In honor of those who care" *Perspectives* 4, no 2 (1999): 3.

Chapter 25: Creating and Communicating With Your Healthcare Team

1. P. Alderton, "Living positively with Alzheimer's." *Early Alzheimer's – A Forum for Early-Stage Dementia Care*, Santa Barbara: Alzheimer's Association, Spring, 1998: 4.

2. R. Ray, "Joan Cahill on Living with Alzheimer's," *NurseWeek.com*. November 7, 2003. www.nurseweek.com/5min/cahill_print.html. Nurse Week Publishing, Inc.

3. G. Sterin, "Prologue," In P. Harris (Ed), *The Person with Alzheimer's Disease*, Baltimore: Johns Hopkins University Press, 2002: xxxiv.

Chapter 26: Helpful Legal and Financial Planning

1. L. Snyder, *Speaking Our Minds–What it's Like to Have Alzheimer's (Revised Edition)*, Baltimore: Health Professions Press, 2009: 117.

2. S. Goldfein, "Speaking Out! Sharing the Experience of Alzheimer's" *Early Alzheimer's-An International Newsletter on Dementia* 4, no 1 (2001): 8.

3. L. Feinberg, C. Whitlach, *Making Hard Choices: Respecting Both Voices*, San Francisco: Family Caregiver Alliance, 2000.

Chapter 27: Maintaining Ongoing Quality of Life

1. R. Logsdon, "Making the Most of Every Day–Quality of Life" In P. Harris (Ed) *The Experience of Alzheimer's*, Baltimore: Johns Hopkins University Press, 2002: 75-87.

2. D. Morhardt, "Top 10 ideas for enhancing quality of life by diagnosed individuals and families living with Alzheimer's disease and related dementias," *Alzheimer's Care Quarterly* 5, no 2 (2004):103-107.

3. *What Happens Next? – A booklet about being diagnosed with Alzheimer's disease or a related disorder.* National Institutes of Health Publication No: 07-6199, October, 2008: 4.

4. R. Litterland, "London develops new early stage program," *Early Alzheimer's* 4, no 1 (2001): 4.

5. Alzheimer's Australia, "Tips for carers from those with memory disorders," *Nest–A Newsletter of Alzheimer's Australia* 7, no 1 (March, 2005).

6. Alzheimer's Association, *Alzheimer's Disease Inside Looking Out.* A video production. Cleveland, OH: Cleveland Area Chapter, 1995.

7. Rush Alzheimer's Disease Newsletter, Chicago, IL: Rush Presbyterian St Luke's Medical Center. Winter, 1993: 6.

8. D. Morhardt, "Top 10 ideas for enhancing quality of life by diagnosed individuals and families living with Alzheimer's disease and related dementias," *Alzheimer's Care Quarterly* 5, no 2 (2004): 105.

9. P. Harris, C. Durkin, "Building resilience through coping and adapting," In P. Harris (Ed) *The Experience of Alzheimer's*, Baltimore: Johns Hopkins University Press, 2002: 174.

10. *Enhancing Wellness – An inspirational guide for people like us with early-stage memory loss - A By Us For Us Guide,* Waterloo, Ontario: Murray Alzheimer's Research and Education Program, University of Waterloo, 2008: 2.

11. P. Reed, S. Bluethmann, *Voices of Alzheimer's Disease–A Summary Report on the Nationwide Town Hall*

Meetings for People with Early Stage Dementia, Chicago, IL: Alzheimer's Association, 2008: 26.
12. L. Snyder, "Brainstorming – Staying Young at Heart" *Perspectives – A Newsletter for Individuals with Alzheimer's or a Related Disorder* 14, no 1 (2008): 4.

Chapter 28: Progress and Trends in Treatment and Care

1. L. Clare, "We'll fight it as long as we can - Coping with the onset of Alzheimer's disease." *Aging and Mental Health* 6, no 2 (2002): 143.
2. L. Snyder, *Speaking Our Minds–What it's Like to Have Alzheimer's (Revised Edition),* Baltimore: Health Professions Press, 2009: 124.
3. T. Kitwood, *Dementia Reconsidered: The Person Comes First,* Buckingham, England: Open University Press, 1997.
4. V. Bell, D. Troxel, *The Best Friend's Approach to Alzheimer's Care,* Baltimore: Health Professions Press, 2003.

Chapter 30: Research Brings Hope For the Future

1. E. Robinson, "Should people with Alzheimer's disease take part in research?" In: H. Wilkinson (Ed). *The Perspective of People with Alzheimer's Disease: Research Methods and Motivations,* London: Jessica Kingsley Publishers, 2002: 104.
2. V. DiMeo, "Finding meaning in Alzheimer's," *Perspectives – A Newsletter for Individuals with Alzheimer's or a Related Disorder* 9, no 1 (2003): 2.
3. B. Shapiro, B Shapiro, "A life beyond diagnosis," *The Massachusetts Chapter of the Alzheimer's Association Newsletter,* Fall, 2003.

✣ Index

A

Acupuncture as treatment, 253
Adolescents
   relationship with, 53-54
   young-onset and, 61-62
Advocacy
   educating elected officials, 166-167
   importance of, 163-165
   public awareness and, 45
   questions for discussion, 170
   reducing stigma through, 236-237
   suggestions, 170
   types of, 168-170
   young-onset and, 64
Age
   disease development and, 14
   memory loss and, 30
Ageless Designs Alzheimer's News Service, 22
Alcohol consumption, 187
Alternative therapies
   acupuncture, 253
   aromatherapy, 252
   brain boosters, 250-251
   creative arts, 253-264
   defined, 247
   metals, 251-252
   nutritional and herbal supplements, 249-250
   questions for discussion, 254-255
   suggestions for being informed consumer, 255
   vitamins or mineral supplements, 247-248
Aluminum, 251
Alzheimer, Alois, 16
Alzheimer Disease International (ADI), 167-168
Alzheimer's Association
   Advisory Group of People with Dementia, 166
   contacting, 22, 212
   services of, 212
Alzheimer's Disease Centers, 211, 264
Alzheimer's Disease Cooperative Study, 264
Alzheimer's Disease Education and Referral (ADEAR)
   contacting, 22, 212
   research participation and, 264
   services of, 212
Alzheimer's Foundation of America
   contacting, 22, 212-213
   services of, 22, 212-213
Americans with Disabilities Act, 59
Amnesia. *See* Memory loss
Anger
   of care partners, 201
   managing, 124-125
   provokers of, 123-124
   as reaction to diagnosis, 26
Anomia, 74-75
Antioxidants, 186
Anxiety
   of care partners, 201
   managing, 125-126
Aphasia, 34
   See also Communication
Apolipoprotein E (APOE), 14-15
Apraxia, 91-92
Aromatherapy, 252
ARTZ: Artist for Alzheimer's, 254
Assistance, accepting. *See* Help, accepting
Assistive technology, 244-245
At the Crossroads, 111
Attitude(s)
   developing and maintaining positive, 130-132, 234-235
   feeling and maintaining hope, 194-196
   importance of, 82
Attorneys, finding, 227-228

B

Best Friends Approach, 243-244
Bill paying, 114-115
Blaming others, 126-128
Body language, 78
Brain boosters, 250-251
Brain fitness programs, 181-183
Brain imaging, 256-257
Brain scans, 17

C

The Calm Before the Storm, 103
Cardiovascular disease, 185-186
Caregivers. *See* Care partners

Care managers, benefits of, 118
Care partners
    feelings of, 200-202
    helping your, 205-206
    medical appointments and, 219
    needs of, 204-205
    questions for discussion, 207
    suggestions for taking care of, 207-208
    support groups and, 136, 137-138, 202-203
    time out for, 203-204
Causes, 14-15
Children
    relationship with, 53-54
    young-onset and, 61-62
Cholesterol, 185-186
Circadian rhythms, 91
Clinical trials, 259-263, 264
Clinical Trials.Gov, 264
Clothing
    dressing self strategies, 92
    keeping, clean, 116
Clutter, dealing with, 100
Coenzyme Q 10 as treatment, 249
Coffee, 187-188
Cognitive training programs, 181-183
Cold weather cautions, 102
Comfort Zone, 87
Communication
    assistance from others, 73-74, 75, 76, 79
    disappearance of words, 74-75
    including patient in, 77
    keeping track of discussions, 75-76
    with members of healthcare team, 219-221
    memory loss and, 72-77
    questions for discussion, 78
    suggestions for improving, 78-79
Community resources
    locating, 212-213
    questions for discussion, 214
    in rural areas, 213
    suggestions for using, 214
    types available, 210-211
Companion role, 147-148
Complementary therapies
    acupuncture, 253
    aromatherapy, 252
    brain boosters, 250-251
    creative arts, 253-264
    defined, 247

    metals, 251-252
    nutritional and herbal supplements, 249-250
    questions for discussion, 254-255
    suggestions for being informed consumer, 255
    vitamins or mineral supplements, 247-248
Conservators, described, 226-228
Control
    fear of loss of, 24-25
    maintaining most longest, 236
Conversations, 33-34
Cooking strategies, 99-100
Coordination and exercise, 173-174
Co-workers, telling about diagnosis, 45-47
Creative arts as treatment, 253-264

D

Dehydration, 102
Dementia
    alcohol consumption and, 187
    Alzheimer's diagnosis and, 16-17
Denial
    by family or friends, 43-44, 48-49
    as reaction to diagnosis, 23-26
    of young-onset, 58-59
Dental fillings, 251
Depression
    exercise and, 172-173
    overcoming, 123-124
    as symptom, 121-122
    weight and, 188
Devastation, feelings of, 27-28
DHA as treatment, 249
Diagnosis
    coming to terms with, 131-132, 135-136
    early, 256-257
    elements of dignified, 18-20
    management techniques for reactions to, 29
    methods of, 16-17
    questions for discussion about telling others, 47
    questions for discussion after, 29
    reactions to, 23-29
    response of family to, 43-44, 48-49
    response of friends to, 43-44, 68-69
    suggestions for discussing with others, 47
    telling family about, 41-43
    telling friends about, 41-43, 67-68
    telling workplace about, 45-47
    value of early, 13

of young-onset, 58-59
Discouragement, 121-123
Disorientation
    in familiar places, 36
    strategies for avoiding, 87-88
Dressing self strategies, 92
Driving
    accidents, 105
    coping with loss of, 108-110, 111
    effect of Alzheimer's on, 104-105
    legal liability, 108
    questions for discussion, 110-111
    state laws and, 106
    when to stop, 107-108
Durable power of attorney, described, 225-226
Durable power of attorney for healthcare,
    described, 226

E

Early onset. *See* Young-onset
Early retirement, 59-61
Eden Alternative, 243
Elder Locator, contact and service information, 212
Elected officials, educating, 166-167
Emergencies, managing, 116-117
Employment and diagnosis, 45-47
Essential oils as treatment, 252
Executive functioning, 128
Exercise
    benefits of, 171-174
    best types and amount, 174
    getting most out of, 177
    getting motivated, 175-176
    pets and, 159
    for physically disabled, 174-175
    questions for discussion, 176-177
Expectations of self, 82

F

Faces, forgetting, 85-87
Faith, 196-197
Falls, preventing, 97-99
Familiarity, importance of, 235
Family
    adjustments to symptoms by, 49-50
    communication assistance from, 73-74, 75, 76, 79
    response to diagnosis by, 43-44, 48-49

risk factors, 14-15, 57-58
shifts in responsibilities and roles, 50-54
strategies for remembering individuals, 85-87
suggestions for strengthening relationships
    with, 54-55
suggestions for young-onset, 65
telling about diagnosis, 41-43
young-onset and, 61-62
Family Caregiver Alliance, contact and service
    information, 212
Feelings
    accepting help and, 142-143
    anger or irritability, 123-125
    anxiety or fright, 125-126
    of care partners, 200-202
    depression or discouragement, 121-123
    developing positive attitudes, 130-132, 234-235
    hope, 194-196
    memory and, 32
    questions for discussion, 132, 199
    of reduced motivation, 128-130
    suggestions for managing, 132, 199
    support groups and, 134-135, 136
    suspiciousness, 126-128
Finances
    managing, 114-115
    memory loss and, 223-224
Financial planning
    for long-term care expenses, 229-230
    need for early, 223-224
    Social Security and disability benefits, 228-229
    veteran's benefits, 230
    of young-onset, 59-61
Fisher Center for Alzheimer's Research Foundation,
    264
Folate supplements, 148
Food and nutrition
    antioxidants and, 186
    cholesterol and, 185-186
    coffee and, 187-188
    food preparation and, 113
    making most of meals, 189-190
    omega-2 fatty acids and, 186-187
    questions for discussion, 190
    suggestions for good, 190-191
Food preparation, managing, 113
Forgetfulness, 32-33
Free legal aid, 227-228
Free radicals, 186-187

Friends
    adjustments to symptoms by, 49-50
    communication assistance from, 73-74, 75, 76, 79
    finding age peers with Alzheimer's, 62-63
    help or support from, 68
    importance of, 151-152
    loss of, as reaction to diagnosis, 68-69
    making new, 69-70, 71
    response to diagnosis by, 43-44
    size of gatherings, 76-77
    strategies for remembering individuals, 85-87
    suggestions for maintaining, 71
    suggestions for strengthening relationships with, 54-55
    telling about diagnosis, 41-43, 67-68
Fright
    diagnosis and, 27-28
    managing, 125-127
Frontotemporal Dementia, 18

G

Genetics
    disease development and, 14-15
    young-onset and, 57-58
Gingko biloba as treatment, 249
Grandchildren, relationship with, 53-54
Gratitude, expressing to care partners, 206-207
Grooming, managing, 115-116
Guardians, described, 226-228

H

Healthcare proxies
    described, 226
    with physician, 222
Healthcare teams
    appointment companion, 219
    appointment preparation, 218-219
    communicating effectively with, 219-221
    neuropsychologists, 217
    nurses and physician assistants, 217
    physicians, 216-217
    purpose of, 215-216
    questions for discussion, 221
    social workers, 218
    suggestions for making most of, 221-222

Help, accepting
    feeling about, 52, 142-143
    as gradual process, 145-146
    helping others by, 148
    independence and, 146
    questions for discussion, 149
    role of personal assistant or companion, 147-148
    signs of need for, 144-145
    suggestions for, 149
Helping others, 149, 160-161
Herbal supplements as treatment, 249-250
Hobbies, developing and maintaining, 153-154
Holidays, enjoying, 157-158
Home
    care managers and staying in, 118
    evaluating living alone, 113-118
    improving safety in, 97-101, 103
    living with someone else in your, 119-120
    maintenance, 117
    managing emergencies, 113
Home Safety for People with Alzheimer's, 103
Hope, feeling and maintaining, 194-196, 199
Hot weather cautions, 102
House keys, 101
Humor, sense of, 192-194, 199
Huperzine A as treatment, 249-250
Hygiene, managing, 115-116
Hypothermia, 102

I

Impatience of care partners, 201-202
Impotency, 38
Independence
    accepting help and, 146
    fear of loss of, 24-25
    suggestions for maintaining, 236
    transition to teamwork from, 51-53
Individuals, recognizing, 35
Information
    sources, 21-22
    storing and retrieving, 29-31
International advocacy, 167-168
Intimacy, 38
Irritability, 123-125
Items, strategies for remembering placement of, 84-85

L

Last wills and testaments, described, 225
Legal planning
  basics, 224-227
  finding attorneys, 227-228
  free, 227-228
  need for early, 223-224
Lewy Body Dementia, 18
Limitations, acceptance of, 235
Living alone
  considering other arrangements, 119-120
  evaluating, 113-118
  questions for discussion, 120
  suggestion for, 120
Living trusts, described, 225
Long-term care, innovative approaches to, 242-244
Long-term care planning
  financial, 59-61, 223-230
  legal, 223-228
  questions for discussion, 231
  suggestions for next steps, 231
Lost, strategies for preventing getting, 87-88
Love, expressing to care partners, 206

M

Marginalization, feelings of, 27
Media images, 24
Medicaid and long-term care expenses, 229
Medic Alert/Safe Return, 87
Medical foods, 250-251
Medicare
  benefits, 60-61
  long-term care expenses and, 229
Medications
  list of, 219
  managing, 114
  sleep and, 90-91
  treatment with approved, 239-240
  weight and, 188
Memories, recording, 155
Memories in the Making, 253-264
Memory loss
  aging and, 30
  communication and, 72-74, 72-77
  diagnosis denial and, 25-26
  disorientation and, 36
  financial/legal matters and, 223-224

intimacy and sexuality and, 38
  mental stimulation and, 178
  of new vs. old information, 31
  reasons for, 16
  suspiciousness and, 127
  symptoms, 32-35
Memory loss management
  cooking strategies, 99-100
  developing own strategies, 89
  general principles, 81-82
  questions for discussion, 88
  strategies for preventing getting disoriented or lost, 87-88
  strategies for remembering names and people, 85-87
  strategies for remembering where you put things, 84-85
  strategies for staying organized, 83-84
Memory processes explained, 31, 32
Mental status tests, 17
Mental stimulation
  doing what you enjoy, 183-184
  importance of, 178
  making most of abilities, 178-179
  paying attention, 180
  questions for discussion, 184
  social activities and, 180-181
  suggestions for, 184
  thinking strategies, 179-180
Mercury, 251
Metals as treatment, 251-252
Mild Cognitive Impairment, 18
Mineral supplements as treatment, 247-248
Mood
  changes, 37
  exercise and, 172-173
  hope, 194-196
Motivation, managing reduced, 128-130
Motor vehicle accidents, 105
Movies, 154-155

N

Names, strategies for remembering, 85-87
National Academy of Elder Law Attorneys, 227
National Alzheimer's Association Advocacy and Public Policy Office, 170
National Association of Professional Geriatric Care Managers, 118

National Do Not Call List, 115
National Library for the Blind and Physically Handicapped, 93
Neuritic plaques, role of, 16
Neurofibrillary tangles, role of, 16
Neurologists, 216
Neuropsychologists, 217
New experiences, 236
News sources, 22
Nurses, 217
Nutraceuticals, 250
Nutrition
    antioxidants and, 186
    cholesterol and, 185-186
    coffee and, 187-188
    food preparation and, 113
    making most of meals, 189-190
    omega-2 fatty acids and, 186-187
    questions for discussion, 190
    suggestions for good, 190-191
Nutritional supplements as treatment, 249-250

O

Omega-2 fatty acids, 186-187
On the tip of the tongue, 74
Organization, maintaining sense of, 235
Organized, strategies for staying, 83-84, 100
Outings, discovering local, 158-159

P

Paraphasic errors, 74
Partnering With Your Doctor: A Guide for Persons with Memory Problems and Their Care Partners, 222
Paying attention, importance of, 180
Peers, finding age peers with Alzheimer's, 62-63
People, recognizing, 35
Perceptual abilities, 35
Personal assistant role, 147-148
Personal health, importance of, 234
Personal hygiene, managing, 115-116
Person-centered care, 242-243
Perspectives: A Newsletter for Individual's with Alzheimer's or a Related Disorder, 22
Pets, 179
Physical activity
    benefits of, 171-174
    best types and amount, 174
    getting most out of, 177
    getting motivated, 175-176
    pets and, 159
    for physically disabled, 174-175
    questions for discussion, 176-177
Physically disabled, exercise for, 174-175
Physician assistants, 217
Physicians
    communicating effectively with, 219-221
    give Healthcare Proxy to, 222
    role of, 216-217
Positive attitudes, developing, 130-132, 234-235
Prevention, 258
Principles for a Dignified Diagnosis, 18-20
Programs, specialized, 152-153
Project Lifesaver, 87
Psychiatrists, 216-217

Q

Quality of life
    core principles of, 232-233
    defined, 232
    questions for discussion, 238
    social activities, 233
    suggestions for maintaining and improving, 63-64, 237-238
Questions for discussion
    accepting help, 149
    advocacy, 170
    care partners, 207
    communication, 78
    community resources, 214
    complementary/alternative therapies, 254-255
    diagnosis, 29
    driving, 110-111
    exercise, 176-177
    family relationships, 54
    feelings, 132, 199
    friends, 70
    healthcare teams, 221
    home safety, 103
    living alone, 120
    long-term care planning, 231
    memory loss management, 88
    mental stimulation, 184
    nutrition, 190
    quality of life, 238

research, 263
sense of humor, 199
social activities, 161
support groups, 140-141
symptoms, 40, 95
telling about diagnosis, 47
treatment, 246
young-onset, 65

R

Reading challenges, 36, 93
Receptive aphasia, 76
Recognition of individuals, 35
Related disorders, 17-18
Relationships
    shifts in responsibilities and roles, 50-54
    suggestions for strengthening, 54-55
    young-onset and, 61-62
    See also Family; Friends
Religion, 196-197
Repetition, 33
Research
    clinical trials, 259-263, 264
    in diagnostic methods, 256-257
    new avenues of, 259
    in new treatments, 257-258
    participating in, 259-263, 264
    prevention and, 258
    questions for discussion, 263
    suggestions for learning more about, 263-264
Rest, importance of, 161
Rigidity, 98
Risk factors, 14-15, 57-58
Routine, importance of maintaining, 235
Routine tasks, completing, 34-35

S

Sadness of care partners, 201
Safety
    during exercise, 175
    general precautions, 235
    preventing falls, 97-99
    preventing getting lost, 87-88
    when to stop driving, 107-108
Selenium, 148
Self-expectations, 82
Sexuality, 38

Shame and diagnosis, 26-27
Shock and diagnosis, 27-28
Sleep
    exercise and, 173
    importance of, 82
    managing disrupted, 90-91
    during travel, 157
Smell, diminished sense of, 37
Social activities
    advocacy, 163-165
    discovering local outings, 158-159
    helping others, 160-161
    hobbies, 153-154
    holidays, 157-158
    importance of, 151-152, 233
    mental stimulation from, 180-181
    movies, 154-155
    new experiences, 236
    overcoming obstacles to, 150-151
    questions for discussion, 161
    specialized programs, 152-153
    suggestions for finding, 162
    weight and, 189
Social isolation
    risk, 117-118
    support groups and, 134-135
Social Security, 60, 228-229
Social workers, 218
Sources of information, 21-22
Spatial abilities, 35
Specialized programs, 152-153
Spiritual faith, 196-197
Stigma
    decreasing, 45
    diagnosis and, 26-27
    reducing through advocacy, 236-237
Strength and exercise, 173-174
Stress
    of care partners, 202, 206
    exercise and, 173
    sense of humor and, 192-193
Sundowning, 94-95
Support groups
    benefits of, 134-138, 241-242
    care partners and, 136, 137-138, 202-203
    choosing not to attend, 139-140
    feeling and maintaining hope and, 195-196
    format and structure of, 133-134
    getting the most out of, 141

overcoming reluctance to participate, 138-139

questions for discussion, 140-141

starting, 140

young-onset and, 62, 63

Suspiciousness, managing, 126-128

Symptoms

completing routine tasks, 34-35

diminished sense of smell or taste, 37

disorientation, 36

financial/legal matters and, 223-224

intimacy or sexuality, 38

main, 13

managing, 39, 49-50, 91-96

memory loss, 30-35

mood changes, 37

questions for discussion, 40, 95

reading and writing challenges, 36

spatial and perceptual abilities, 35

understanding, 40

vision changes, 35

See also Memory loss

T

Taste, diminished sense of, 37

Teamwork transition from independence, 51-53

Technology as treatment, 244-245

Teenagers

relationship with, 53-54

young-onset and, 61-62

Tension and exercise, 173

Testing

genetic, 15

mental status, 17

Thinking, stimulating, 179-180

Travel, 156-157

Treatment

acupuncture, 253

aromatherapy, 252

assistive technology, 244-245

brain boosters, 250-251

creative arts, 253-264

education, 241-242

innovative long-term care, 242-244

medications, 239-240

metals, 251-252

nutritional and herbal supplements, 249-250

of other health conditions, 141

questions for discussion, 246, 254-255

research and, 257-258

suggestions for effective participation in, 246

vitamin or mineral supplements, 247-248

See also Support groups

V

Vascular Dementia, 18

Verbal abilities, 33-34

Veteran's benefits, 230

Visual agnosia, 35

Vitamin supplements as treatment, 247-248

W

Weapons, 101

Weather cautions, 102

Weight, 188-189

Wernicke-Korsakoff Syndrome, 187

Withdrawal risk, 117-118

Writing challenges, 36, 94

Y

Young-onset

financial planning and, 59-61

genetic factors and, 14, 57-58

overview of, 56-57

suggestions for families, 65

support groups for, 134

Z

Zinc, 148

Also Available From Sunrise River Press

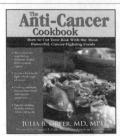

The Anti-Cancer Cookbook
How to Cut Your Risk with the Most Powerful, Cancer-Fighting Foods

by Dr. Julia Greer, MD, MPH Dr. Julia Greer—a physician, cancer researcher, and food enthusiast—explains what cancer is and how antioxidants work to prevent pre-cancerous mutations in your body's cells, and then describes which foods have been scientifically shown to help prevent which types of cancer. She then shares her collection of more than 220 scrumptious recipes for soups, sauces, main courses, vegetarian dishes, sandwiches, breads, desserts, and beverages, all loaded with nutritious ingredients chock-full of powerful antioxidants that may significantly slash your risk of a broad range of cancer types, including lung, colon, breast, prostate, pancreatic, bladder, stomach, leukemia, and others. If you love good food and are looking for delicious ways to keep yourself and your family healthy and cancer-free, you'll find yourself reaching for this book time and again. Softbound, 7.5 x 9 inches, 224 pages. **Item # SRP149**

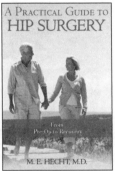

A Practical Guide to Hip Surgery
From Pre-Op to Recovery

M.E. Hecht, MD This book tells you everything you need to know before you undergo hip replacement or resurfacing surgery, directly from an orthopedic surgeon who has performed countless hip surgeries and has undergone a double hip replacement herself! Dr. M.E. Hecht tells you step by step what you'll need to do before the day of your surgery, and then walks you through the procedure itself so that you know exactly what to expect. Sharing from her own experience as a hip surgery patient, she also discusses issues that can arise during the first few days through first months of your recovery, and includes handy checklists to help you organize and plan for your post-surgery weeks so you can focus on recovering as quickly and smoothly as possible. This book is a must-read before you undergo surgery, and will prove to be a trusted and essential resource during and after your hospital stay. Softbound, 6 x 9 inches, 160 pages. **Item # SRP612**

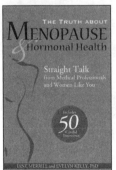

The Truth about Menopause & Hormonal Health
Straight Talk from Medical Professionals and Women Like You

With the advent of bioidentical hormones and the controversies surrounding synthetic hormones, many women are confused about whether hormone therapy is safe. Women are increasingly empowered about their health and want the best advice and information available. Rather than promote a specific hormone therapy, The Truth about Menopause & Hormonal Health provides an objective survey of the treatments available from the conservative to the alternative end of the spectrum. You'll find experience-based help and good medical sense in The Truth about Menopause & Hormonal Health. The pros and cons of all types of hormone therapies – synthetic, plant-based, bioidentical, and alternative – are discussed in detail. Insightful interviews with women and healthcare professionals are part of each discussion. These perspectives help clear up the confusion about what's necessary for hormonal health and help you make your own decision to suit your lifestyle. Softbound, 6 x 9 inches, 176 pages. **Item # SRP636**

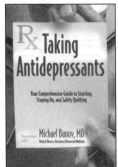

Taking Antidepressants
Your Comprehensive Guide to Starting, Staying On, and Safely Quitting

Michael Banov, MD Antidepressants are the most commonly prescribed class of medications in this country. Yet, consumers have few available resources to educate them about starting and stopping antidepressants. Dr. Michael Banov walks the reader through a personalized process to help them make the right choice about starting antidepressants, staying on antidepressants, and stopping antidepressants. Readers will learn how antidepressant medications work, what they may experience while taking them, and will learn how to manage side effects or any residual or returning depression symptoms. Softbound, 6 x 9 inches, 304 pages. **Item # SRP606**